TRADITIONAL CHINESE MEDICINE
A Natural Guide to Weight Loss That Lasts

Also by Nan Lu, O.M.D., L.Ac., with Ellen Schaplowsky

Traditional Chinese Medicine:
A Woman's Guide to Healing from Breast Cancer

TRADITIONAL CHINESE MEDICINE
A Natural Guide to Weight Loss That Lasts

NAN LU, O.M.D., M.S., L.AC.,
with Ellen Schaplowsky

Quill
An Imprint of HarperCollins*Publishers*

The Dragon's Way™ is a registered trademark.

TRADITIONAL CHINESE MEDICINE: A NATURAL GUIDE TO WEIGHT LOSS THAT LASTS. Copyright © 2000 by Dr. Nan Lu. All rights reserved. Printed in the United States of America. No part of this book may be used or reproduced in any manner whatsoever without written permission except in the case of brief quotations embodied in critical articles and reviews. For information address HarperCollins Publishers Inc., 10 East 53rd Street, New York, NY 10022.

HarperCollins books may be purchased for educational, business, or sales promotional use. For information please write: Special Markets Department, HarperCollins Publishers Inc., 10 East 53rd Street, New York, NY 10022.

FIRST EDITION

Designed by Rhea Braunstein

Library of Congress Cataloging-in-Publication Data has been applied for.

ISBN 0-380-80905-2

00 01 02 03 04 RRD 10 9 8 7 6 5 4 3 2

*To my many extraordinary masters who have
gifted me with the deep knowledge and spirit
of true healing.*

*To my family—my parents and sisters,
my wife, Ling Shou, and my children,
Christina and Alicia.*

NAN LU

*To Nan Lu for his extraordinary ability
to create light wherever he goes;
To my son, Ian, my sister, Pat, and brothers
Michael, Tom, Jim, and Peter;
to my extended family, dear friends, and
Qigong sisters and brothers.*

ELLEN H. SCHAPLOWSKY

Contents

Foreword

How Do I Know If The Dragon's Way™ Is for Me?

*H*ᴀᴠᴇ you been on many diets? No matter how hard you try, do you always regain the weight you take off? Do you regain even more weight after a diet? Have you tried again and again to lose weight yet can't seem to achieve satisfying results? Are you puzzled about your extra weight, because you really don't feel that you overeat? Is it always those last few pounds that cause you to become unbelievably frustrated? Do you have certain health conditions (such as migraines, indigestion, etc.) that you've been told, or you suspect, are linked to your excess weight? Then The Dragon's Way should become your way. This is the program that can offer you a healthy way to get off the weight loss merry-go-round—a way that you can use for the rest of your life.

We urge you to put aside all your preconceptions about diets and dieting before you read this book. The Dragon's Way is unlike any other "diet" program you have been on or heard about. In fact, it isn't really a "diet program" as you have come to know it in the Western world. Yet, if you follow The Dragon's Way, you will find that weight will come off. You will also discover something remarkable. Once you have helped your body rebalance itself and helped your five major organ systems (liver, heart, spleen, lung, and kidney) to work in harmony again, you can pretty much eat whatever you want! (Well, no, you can't have chocolate cake for breakfast every other day and a sixteen-ounce steak for dinner every night of your life. But, you won't even want to.) The Dragon's Way will help you learn how to think about food in a whole new way. A way that is healing and healthy for your body. In fact, most often you won't have to think about or obsess about food any more, which many former dieters tell us is a big relief. Your body will let you know what it needs naturally. And perhaps for the first time ever, you'll be able to hear what your body wants and respond to its needs in a healthful manner.

How can this be? The Dragon's Way is unique. It's about two things that you will not find in virtually any Western diet program or product: It's about Qi, or vital energy, your life force, and it's about reawakening the ability to heal yourself. This program is based on the ancient principles of traditional Chinese medicine (TCM), one of the oldest holistic medical systems in the world.

TCM is not New Age medicine. Nor is it a basket full of different techniques. It has been in continuous use for more than five thousand years, keeping millions upon millions of individuals healthy for thousands of years. Today TCM is thriving in China. It is practiced side by side and has equal status with Western medicine in China's top hospitals, teaching colleges and medical centers as a well-respected healing modality. It is time-tested medicine that is just now being understood and recognized throughout the world for the tremendous benefits it can bring.

"Self-healing" can mean many things to many people. In TCM, it means awakening or recalling the body's own inborn healing ability, a talent which everyone has, and reconnecting the internal dots so that all your systems function at their best in three ways: first in and of themselves, second with each other, and third with the Universe itself, the very ancient web into which TCM believes all things are woven. The key to powering your organs' systems is Qi. In the case of The Dragon's Way, this amazing healing restoration is accomplished with *Wu Ming* Meridian Therapy, a special ancient self-healing Qigong practice that you will learn and practice daily. This can be done anywhere, anytime by just about anyone.

Most Western people who read this book will immediately read the list of recommended foods to see what kind of a "diet" The Dragon's Way offers. I urge you not to do that. Otherwise you will completely miss the most powerful and the most effective part of this program, *Wu Ming* Meridian Therapy. This is the secret key to our program and Dr. Lu's gift to you. It is the real answer to weight gain and weight retention. By learning the meridian stretches in the Qigong movements, you can take off or "give up" your excess weight and inches. Most importantly, you can heal the root cause of your weight problems. You'll feel better than you ever thought you could. You'll feel better because you *are* better! Dr. Lu deliberately avoids using the term "lose weight." He says, "What happens when you lose something? You try to get it back. In the case of extra weight, you don't want it back! You want it gone for good. Thoughts are very powerful and suggesting to yourself daily that you are *giving up* extra weight can help you substantially in this program."

Before you go any further, take a moment to answer the following questions. You may find some of these questions unusual for a "diet" book, but these are typical questions a practitioner of TCM would ask you. Why? The answers will speak volumes about the true state of your body's health and will help you to understand which organs are out of balance and in need of healing. When these organs are rebalanced, or their normal healthy function is restored, weight begins to drop off naturally. By the time you complete The Dragon's Way plan as it is outlined in this book, you will have the knowledge you need to understand how your body really works and how to address the fundamental factors that have caused your body to put on or retain excess weight. We think you will be very surprised at the answers. Much of this is information that you probably have never heard before. You'll also be able to read about the health benefits that almost all Dragon's Way participants have been able to achieve. We believe you can achieve similar benefits too.

How many of the following statements apply to you today?

❏ I have tried several different diets and/or workout programs and have not achieved the results I expected.
❏ Even though I eat a "healthy diet," I can't seem to take off weight.
❏ I find it difficult, if not impossible, to adhere to most diet programs.
❏ I lose weight, only to put it back on again.
❏ I cannot seem to lose weight past a certain point. I can get close to my goal, but those last stubborn pounds just won't go away.
❏ The only way I have ever lost weight was by using some form of appetite suppressant.
❏ I would like to lose weight and inches and be able to maintain a slimmer body without feeling like my whole life is one constant "diet."
❏ When choosing foods to eat, I always think about losing or maintaining a certain weight.
❏ There are times I don't allow myself to eat, even though I may be hungry, because I'm afraid of gaining weight.
❏ I believe that I need rigid rules about food in order to eat well.
❏ I don't have the energy to work out regularly.
❏ I think I have food allergies.
❏ I am sensitive to certain foods.
❏ I crave sweets.
❏ I crave carbohydrates.

- ❏ I have other eating cravings, such as strongly sour or salty foods.
- ❏ I have a "dry mouth" frequently.
- ❏ I am often bloated after eating.
- ❏ I have ongoing digestive problems such as heartburn.
- ❏ I am often either constipated or have diarrhea.
- ❏ I am tired or sleepy after meals.
- ❏ I have trouble sleeping at night.
- ❏ I have headaches shortly after eating.
- ❏ I have headaches at the same time every day.
- ❏ I often wake up with a headache.
- ❏ I often have insomnia.
- ❏ I become tired every afternoon at the same time.
- ❏ I am often groggy when I wake up.
- ❏ I am always tired.
- ❏ I have health complaints that are not related to any specific illness, yet when I go to the doctor, he or she tells me that I am fine.
- ❏ Although I am not "sick," I don't feel really well.
- ❏ I often have premenstrual syndrome (PMS) symptoms.
- ❏ I am experiencing menopausal symptoms.
- ❏ My nails have little or no half moons showing.
- ❏ My nails are always brittle or break easily.
- ❏ I never seem to have enough energy.
- ❏ I am very susceptible to colds.
- ❏ I worry excessively.
- ❏ I have become increasingly moody and cranky.
- ❏ I have to have coffee every morning to "get going."
- ❏ I would like to stop smoking, but I don't have the "energy" I need when I don't smoke.
- ❏ I would definitely gain weight if I stopped smoking.
- ❏ My life has gotten too stressful for me.
- ❏ I struggle every day to maintain my weight.
- ❏ Thinking about food and what I should and shouldn't eat takes up an enormous part of my mental activity.

❏ When I think about my weight, I feel frustrated or defeated.

❏ I often feel like a "diet failure."

If you have checked off more than three of these statements, we can honestly say that The Dragon's Way can help you make some wonderful changes in your life, your weight, the way you deal with the nourishment that goes into your body, and the healthy choices you can make each day to live a long, healthy life. With his unique knowledge of TCM and his profound understanding of Qi, the true secret behind TCM, Dr. Lu is offering you the gift of a lifetime. And, the good news is that it is a gift that will last you a lifetime. We believe that this book will be the best investment in your health that you will ever make. So please read on . . .

Ellen H. Schaplowsky
Vice President
Traditional Chinese Medicine World Foundation

Introduction

Eastern Perspective on a Serious Western Health Condition

*B*EFORE you begin this book, there is something important I would like to share with you: whether you are a woman or a man; an adult or a teenager; whether you have been on one diet or dozens; whether you have ten pounds to lose or more than one hundred—you will not permanently solve your weight problem until you fix its underlying root cause. It is as simple (and as complex) as that. Virtually all Western weight loss programs and products address the symptoms, not the source, of excess weight or weight retention. With The Dragon's Way, you have at last discovered a program that can get to the bottom of this health condition.

The information I am about to provide is not a new concept that I invented yesterday. It is not a marketing program promoting some commercial product that you must take for a very long time. It is based on the time-tested philosophy, theories and techniques of traditional Chinese medicine (TCM). This holistic medical system has been in *continuous* practice for many thousands of years. Today, TCM is alive and well in China and around the world.

TCM is just now becoming more widely known in the

United States, where there are more than fifteen thousand licensed professionals in thirty-seven states practicing acupuncture, one of its more popular and better-known healing methods. Today there are sixty-five colleges of TCM that teach TCM theories and acupuncture and are graduating more than fifteen hundred new acupuncturists yearly. Perhaps two of the most important events supporting the efficacy of acupuncture are: the World Health Organization (WHO) notification of countries worldwide about forty-three specific conditions that this healing method can address effectively, and the National Institutes of Health (NIH) consensus statement on endorsing acupuncture as an effective treatment for nausea caused by chemotherapy and pregnancy, and for pain resulting from surgery as well as a variety of musculoskeletal conditions.

More and more, major insurance companies are offering coverage for acupuncture, acupressure, and TCM herbal therapies. Interestingly, TCM herbs are the fastest growing segment of the herbal remedies category, which is projected to reach $16 billion dollars in retail sales by 2003. This trend of growing consumer interest is noted in Dr. David Eisenberg's study in the November 1998 issue of the *Journal of the American Medical Association,* which describes Americans as embracing alternative or complementary medicine in unprecedented numbers. In it, Eisenberg notes that consumers are taking their search for effective, natural, noninvasive health care very seriously. They are taking it so seriously, in fact, that they are investing more than $27 billion of their own money and making more visits to alternative care providers than to Western primary care practitioners in a one-year period.

TCM is one complementary healing system that is clearly striking a chord with many who are searching for natural ways to remain healthy and prevent illness and disease. I am a doctor of TCM, not a Western doctor with some TCM training. I have been trained in the principles, theories, and technical practices of this ancient medicine. In my practice, I see thousands of patients a year. Approximately 95 percent are Western individu-als. Today, I find more and more people visit my Center because they are searching for natural ways to deal with their health problems and to find a lasting solution. This is particularly true for those who want to take off excess weight. Many try TCM as a last resort, but I believe almost everyone is pleased with the results. Often though, the results are not what they expected when they initiated this process!

My overall task as a TCM practitioner is not to treat just the condition of excess weight. TCM treats the whole person. So, it is critical to form a partnership with each person within which he or she can spark his or her own healing power. How do TCM practitioners do this? This approach differs from that of Western medicine. I like to tell my new patients: "I am not the bus driver. I do not make all the decisions. We must work together so that you can learn how to heal yourself. It is your body and you must take responsibility for healing yourself. My role is to help you and to motivate you and to offer you hope and strength." And, when we talk about healing, we talk about the body, mind, emotions, and spirit, because TCM understands that they are inseparable and each affects the others.

In this book, I will share special ways you can heal yourself from the condition of excess weight. Most importantly, I will help you learn simple, but powerful Qigong energy movements called *Wu Ming* Meridian Therapy. These ancient self-healing movements, or meridian stretches, can increase Qi, open up energy blocks, and prevent Qi stagnation. We'll also spend some time learning how each major organ is influenced by a specific associated emotion, and how an excess of that emotion can liter-ally unbalance or damage the function of that organ. We will discuss what you can do to change your lifestyle and minimize stress as well as anger—both of which can take a deadly toll on your liver function. From my experience, I believe that most individuals in Western culture don't realize the role that stress plays in weight problems. The Dragon's Way will show you why and how it does.

This program is deeply rooted in the principle of prevention. It teaches skills that will enable you to maintain newly gained levels of health. Because you will learn theories and skills you can use for a lifetime, for the intelligent participant there is no time when the program ends. My hope for you is that you will make this a lifelong practice. The last day of your Dragon's Way is its true beginning. These six weeks and preparation week are practice sessions to learn how to integrate the basic ideas and techniques that you can explore and sharpen over time.

Prevention will become your true cure. The natural integration of these principles and tools in your life will enable you to identify what works uniquely for you. When your underlying unbalanced internal conditions have been brought back into balance, you will find that your body will not be vulnerable to creating extra weight. I believe it will be stronger than you have ever experienced. You will also handle stress differently. Your ability to regain your internal balance, should you falter, will be greatly enhanced. With your newly found healing tools, what was once a fall can become just a slight stumble.

By the time you read this book, more than one thousand people will have been through The Dragon's Way program. We have been teaching this program with great success to people of different ages and life experiences for almost five years. When we begin the first class of each program, participants are very focused on food. Nine times out of ten, they want to know, "What can I eat?" "What can't I eat?" "What should I eliminate?" "What should I give up?" Their questions are naturally enough centered around what they've been taught and what they've been exposed to in Western weight loss culture, in which the focus is on an external factor: food. Most have not yet been introduced to the self-healing principles behind The Dragon's Way.

Almost immediately, they seem to express a feeling of temporary deprivation. In other words, they're quite sure they have to "suffer" through The Dragon's Way program and give up the things they love in order to get where they want to be weight-wise. There's usually more than a hint of, "I hope I can live through this and get back to my old life after this is over" in their questions. I have very good news, though, for our participants. I would say that every person who graduates from The Dragon's Way is changed in a favorable, fundamental way that opens his or her eyes, as well as his or her body, mind, emotions, and spirit, to a new way of looking at life and to a deep understanding of how to make healthful healing choices. Above all, I believe what they love about this program is the unfolding realization that they do indeed possess their own healing ability and they can apply it to their weight problems—with excellent results!

Now, when we start the first class, before participants even have a chance to raise the question about which foods they can't eat, I immediately tell them to, "throw away any ideas you've ever had about dieting and weight loss because The Dragon's Way is unlike any program you have ever participated in. In fact," I tell them, "this isn't a diet at all. It's a true self-healing program. And, the simple truth is that a body in balance does not have weight problems. Period. Together our goal is to bring you back into balance so you can eliminate your weight problems for good."

The Dragon's Way is not about food restrictions, appetite suppression, or vigorous exercise. It's about understanding the miraculous complexity and delicacy of your body and the way it really works, about how its five major organ systems should operate in harmony, and how Qi, or vital energy, powers all its functions. You are getting a special gift with this program: the owner's manual for your body. Once you receive this knowledge, you can use it for the rest of your life. The basics don't change because they are in harmony with the way the Universe works. The basics follow nature's law, not man's law, or a company's law; they can never go out of style, nor can they ever steer you wrong. Everything you will learn in this book is a result of an understanding of the time-tested holistic medical theories of TCM: Qi and Blood, Meridian Theory, Yin and Yang Energy Theory, and The Five Element Theory. We have no fads, no "instant miracles"—though Qigong, the ancient self-healing energy system that is the basis of The Dragon's Way, has produced more than its share of modern miracles for many.

When I refer to Qi, I'm not referring to "pep" or stamina, or the kind of mental energy on which most of us in Western society run our lives. I am talking about something vastly different. Qi is the very life force of the Universe. It animates all things—both living and nonliving. It makes up the Sun, the Moon, the Earth, and, of course, human beings! Although Qi is an invisible force, it is as real as wind or gravity or electromagnetics. Often Qi is described as energy, but as you go through The Dragon's Way, it will help you immensely to understand that Qi contains two essential elements: one is power, the other is the special message carried by the power.

Let's see how the concept of Qi can be applied to a body organ that's related to weight problems, the liver. Without the proper level of power, the liver will be too weak to perform its appropriate functions, which are the assigned tasks that it is programmed by nature to accomplish. In TCM, these functions extend beyond the physical to incorporate the emotional and spiritual aspects of the organ as well. Without the proper message, the organ itself will not know what it's supposed to do. Keeping Qi strong, then, plays an essential role in keeping the body's whole complex of interrelated systems humming smoothly and efficiently. When this state is achieved, you either lose weight naturally or maintain a healthy normal weight (not someone else's idea of how much you should weigh). And, you don't have to obsess about food to do this.

From my experience as a TCM practitioner, I believe that

too many people have an unrealistic expectation of what constitutes a healthy weight. I am particularly concerned with the young women I see. They are deeply conditioned by advertising and the media to believe that they are too heavy. Wherever they turn, there are unrealistic pictures of women whom they are supposed to imitate. There are very few representations of normal women of normal weight. Consequently, these young women adopt unhealthy eating and lifestyle habits. And what they don't understand is that these very habits are what will unbalance their organs and cause them to gain weight, thus ensuring that a vicious cycle will continue to run their lives.

As we've said, Qi is the true foundation of TCM; it's also one of the fundamental principles of The Dragon's Way. TCM always considers a person's health in terms of her or his Qi and how weak or strong it is. It works from the fundamental premise that as long as an individual's Qi remains strong and flows freely and the body's organs work in harmony, disease or illness cannot enter—not even cancer! Again, this is not a concept that I invented, but that of the *Nei Jing,* the classical medical text written more than two thousand years ago. The opposite, however, is true as well. If your Qi is weak and stagnating, or not flowing freely, and your body's organs are not working in harmony, disease or illness and conditions of imbalance, such as excess weight, can and do enter.

Here's an analogy that seems to work very well when I describe Qi to my classes. "Think of your body like a car," I tell my Dragon's Way participants. "Both your body and your car need power to run, but the parts inside also have to function well. For your car to operate, it needs gas and a properly functioning engine. All the parts must be there; each part must do what it's designed to do. But also, all the connections among these parts must work harmoniously as well. You could say that the parts need to communicate with each other in a smooth way. Otherwise, even with plenty of gas, your car won't run well." It's the same with your organ systems.

Here's another way to look at this. In some ways, your body is also like a computer. For the computer to function well, you need both software and power. Suppose you have a project that needs several software programs to achieve its goal. With the software, but without power, the computer won't run. Without the software and with power, the computer is still nonfunctional. Different software programs are like different individual organ systems. If the programs cannot communicate with each other, then you will not be able to complete your project.

It is virtually the same with the human body. You must have a certain level of Qi on which your whole body depends to power the organ systems for the tasks of your daily life. And each organ, which has its own function, purpose, and Qi, must work in and of itself and then in harmony with your other organs (just the way the software programs needed to work together). To remain in a state of health, everything in your body must work according to its own design and purpose. Otherwise, imbalances or disharmonies can develop and disease or illness can and do enter. And when TCM talks about disease-producing agents or pathogens, you will be surprised to learn what it considers pathogenic. An excess of just about anything can upset the body's delicate internal gyroscope, even emotions and climate.

One form of disharmony is excess weight. Think about this. Healthy bodies do not suffer from problems of excess weight. Nor are they bone-thin. This makes sense, doesn't it? Most people in the West don't have this concept. Many feel they are "healthy," even though they suffer from frequent headaches, digestive problems, insomnia, vague aches and pains, and of course, excess weight. They accept these conditions as "normal." (Sometimes they medicate themselves and the symptoms may vanish, but they're really just suppressed, not healed.) TCM would disagree and identify all these conditions as symptoms related to a Qi deficiency and a deeper imbalance of one or more organs. And TCM would identify ways to treat these problems at their root cause.

When I began our Dragon's Way program I knew that it could really make a difference in the lives of many individuals who have struggled with weight problems, often for quite a few years. And it has. Now my goal is very simple: I want to share with as many individuals as possible the time-tested medical knowledge that has successfully helped literally millions and millions of Chinese people for many thousands of years and continues to do so today.

I also want to help you understand the TCM perspective of why and how a person gains, retains, and regains weight. This endless negative cycle is definitely not good for you. The Dragon's Way can help you break this cycle once and for all. You can finally get to the root cause of your weight problems. Once you awaken your own natural healing ability through our *Wu Ming* Meridian Therapy Qigong, you will be able to get off the weight loss merry-go-round. I want to help educate you about how to apply this knowledge for your own self-healing. I believe you will be amazed at the results and how well you will feel. This process is not about deprivation: it's about regaining your own vitality and reclaiming your true birthright—a healthy body. Once you have this knowledge, no one can take it away. You will have the healing tools of a lifetime . . . for a lifetime!

Many participants are curious about the program's name and ask me, "Why the Dragon?" I tell them that in history many cultures have magical and mythical beasts. For people of the East, including the Chinese for whom the dragon is their national symbol, the dragon is a magical being. The dragon is a symbol of miraculous things and represents the collective wisdom of Chinese culture, which encompasses not only the art of TCM, but other arts as well such as painting, calligraphy, music, and Feng Shui (the healing art of place and placement), as well as the martial arts, which are healing arts in their original form.

I believe it is an appropriate name for this program. The dragon's way is considered one of wisdom, a way where freedom of body, mind, emotions, and spirit flows. This ancient natural healing wisdom can be yours. My wish is that The Dragon's Way can now become your way. May your journey to good health in a body healed of excess weight be a successful one!

Nan Lu, O.M.D., L.Ac.

TRADITIONAL CHINESE MEDICINE
A Natural Guide to Weight Loss That Lasts

CHAPTER 1
WEIGHT AND HEALTH:
The TCM Perspective

As I mentioned earlier, TCM has been in uninterrupted use for about five thousand years. Its theories are based on a deep understanding of the very essence of nature and the Universe. By applying its principles to the human body, this healing art evolved and was enriched over time.

If you consider the body as a unified and integrated energy system rather than a collection of independent parts, you can begin to appreciate the perspective of TCM, which sees everything woven into one magnificent web of life. When a person comes to a TCM doctor with a complaint, the practitioner looks for the root or energy cause of the imbalance. He or she carefully checks and evaluates the energy systems and treats these root causes with time-tested healing techniques such as special foods, herbs, acupuncture, *Tuina* or acupressure, and moxibustion (the application of heat to acupoints), and even a form of Chinese psychology. All of these are aimed specifically at restoring, rebalancing, and increasing the Qi of an affected organ or organs and helping Qi flow smoothly through the meridians, invisible channels that form the body's energy network.

When TCM discusses the function of an organ, it is always

1

in the context of its Qi and in relation to the other organ(s) with which it must share a cooperative relationship. For example, if you have chronic constipation, TCM would not rely on treating the symptoms with laxatives or fiber. Rather, TCM would explore the root cause, and for every person, the root cause can be different. For instance, teenage constipation and adult constipation may be treated in two entirely different ways. A number of women experience constipation before their periods. This too would require different treatment. For TCM, your constipation may be related not only to your large intestine, but perhaps your gallbladder, your liver, your stomach, or even your lung. So you see, what may appear to be a large intestine problem—like constipation—may actually arise from a Qi deficiency in the function of other organs. What does this mean? It means that one or more of the involved organs' Qi is too low or too weak to cooperate with the large intestine and help it perform its job of ridding the body of waste material. You can see then why over-the-counter remedies can only treat the symptoms, not the source. If they could treat the source, those who suffer from a recurring problem such as constipation wouldn't have to take these remedies repeatedly for many years.

At the heart of TCM is the tenet that its practitioners must always look for and then treat the root cause of the imbalances that create symptoms of disease. Using modern day terminology, TCM is holistic in its approach. It views every aspect of your life, body, mind, emotions, and spirit as part of the same circle rather than separate, loosely connected pieces to be dealt with individually as if they were only peripherally related to each other. Thus, according to TCM, excess weight is considered a symptom, albeit an important symptom, of a greater health issue, and not the true issue itself. And, you can readily see from this philosophy that once the root cause has been corrected, then the issue has truly been resolved, not simply suppressed, or covered up waiting for a chance to reemerge. In the case of weight problems, I have seen this ever-present burden of excess weight finally lifted from many people who have tried their best to address their weight problems and failed because they did not know about "treating the root cause," the first TCM principle.

Most likely, if you've been on many diets, you've been conditioned to believe that the weight is the problem, that the calories are the problem, or that not enough exercise is the problem. TCM believes that the answer lies *inside* your body itself, not outside. TCM says that excess weight is an external symptom of a deeper imbalance between different organs such as the spleen and the liver, which, in turn, cause problems with an individual's Qi, or energy. If you came to me as a patient with a weight problem, I would recognize this as a red flag signaling deeper health issues. By treating the underlying condition as diagnosed by TCM principles, we would begin to see your weight drop off naturally. I cannot emphasize this enough: TCM believes *weight problems are symptoms of other imbalances that must be healed and not the problem itself.*

This makes sense when you think about the statistics of weight programs and products. Have you ever wondered why it is that 95 percent of all successful dieters regain some or all of their lost weight? People try so hard to take off weight and inches, yet most of them are not going to have permanent success. It's because the underlying problems are still there. Only by healing the root cause can long-lasting results be obtained. This is a very powerful and important concept and the premise of The Dragon's Way. Here's an individual who learned the value of treating the root cause.

When I retired from teaching last year, I expected that my anxiety and muscle tension would end. Instead, I found that I had a stubborn case of high blood pressure. I decided that I didn't want to take medication for my nervousness and my doctor thought if I lost weight, my blood pressure might go down as well. This was important to me because I also didn't want to take blood pressure medication. I didn't know any-

*thing about TCM when I signed up for The Dragon's Way,
but it sounded interesting. For the very first time ever, I was
able to adhere to a program for six weeks. Practicing the* Wu
Ming *Meridian Therapy increased my* Qi, *or energy. I never
realized that my inability to stick to a Western weight loss
program, tension and anxiety were products of low energy. I
never recognized that I had low energy because I was so
conditioned to push myself even when I was fatigued. The
worst part of all is that I didn't understand that I was
ignoring my body's own signals to slow down. I gave up
twenty-three pounds and a whole slew of physical symptoms.
My high blood pressure changed significantly as well. I'm
fifty-five and my life is just beginning!*

PATRICIA B., 55-YEAR-OLD COLLEGE PROFESSOR

TCM'S UNDERSTANDING OF THE MOST COMMON CAUSES OF EXCESS WEIGHT

Mucus and the Spleen

TCM recognizes several causes of excess weight; one is a
mucus problem. Surprising? Mucus is a substance that can occur
anywhere in the body and can be caused by a number of things.
Sometimes mucus can be the result of a dietary issue—too many
dairy products, particularly heavy cheeses, are known to be
mucus-producing. When excess mucus is a dietary matter, TCM
says that there is almost always a dysfunction in a person's lung
or spleen. When we speak about a lung or spleen problem, TCM
means that the physical organs themselves may be all right, but
the way they are functioning, or performing their ingrained
tasks, is not. TCM states that the spleen is the organ/mechanism
that produces mucus; the lung is the organ that stores it. These
activities are part of their normal functions. If either or both
of these organs are malfunctioning, many problems can occur,
including excess weight. It may be that this is the root cause of

your weight problem. If so, unless you restore the relationship between these two organs, it is unlikely that you will be able to take off the weight you want or keep it off.

On the other hand, excess mucus can also result from something else: a person's lifestyle. That seems strange, doesn't it? Without an understanding of TCM and its holistic medical framework, there is no way for you to know how important this statement is. The real health-robbing villain of the turn of the twentieth century (and the millennium) in our frenetic Western culture is stress. Stress creates a negative vibration that can literally unbalance liver function. Stress can easily compromise the liver's ability to function properly and smoothly, which, in turn, causes the spleen and the whole digestive system to become unbalanced. The reason is that the liver and spleen must work as partners to keep your digestive system running well. In this case, TCM would trace the root cause of excess mucus to your liver. Having a problem with one organ is sometimes like a game of dominoes: sooner or later the other organs will fall as well.

Water and the Lung, Spleen, and Kidney

Another excess weight-causing factor that TCM recognizes is excess water in the body. If that is the case, then three key interrelated organs—the lung, spleen, and kidney—are suffering from a function problem. According to TCM, all three play a role in the metabolism and workings of water within the body. The lung maintains control of water in the upper body, the spleen maintains control in the middle, and the kidney monitors water in the lower. For your body to eliminate water when it should, each of these three major organs must function properly in and of themselves. That would seem to be self-evident. But that's not their only function; each must have a harmonious relationship with the other two organs. This triangular partnership must work smoothly. If it doesn't or can't, then you will definitely retain water. And while you can take diuretics to rid yourself of excess water and gain some temporary relief, step back and ask yourself, "Can I take diuretic pills forever? Have I really treated the root cause?" You can also see why diuretics fail to work some of the time. They can only address one aspect of water retention, when there are really three.

Digestion: A Holistic Function

Most people in Western cultures are fairly well educated on the digestive function from the scientific perspective. Certainly, there is a lot of advertising for products that address various aspects of stomach distress and other stomach problems. The TCM view of digestion is broader and more holistic. It views digestion as a whole body function. That is, your body should be able to process smoothly and eventually let go of everything that enters it—not only food, but emotions as well.

This is a critical concept, especially in The Dragon's Way. Why? Because in its Five Element Theory TCM recognizes that each of the five major organs—liver, heart, spleen, lung, and kidney—has a ruling emotion: anger, happiness, worry or overthinking, sadness, and fear, respectively. If you experience these emotions and they remain "stuck" or undigested in your body, Qi cannot move freely through your organs and their meridians and they will become clogged. The result? You will gain or retain excess weight. As you'll see, The Dragon's Way *Wu Ming* Meridian Therapy directly addresses this problem.

I'd like to share some insights that I have discovered over many years of working with Western patients. Almost all of the overweight people that I deal with eat fairly well. They seldom eat a lot of junk food; many are vegetarians or eat organic foods; their eating habits are fairly healthy. For some people, what you eat and how you eat can cause digestive system problems. Those are external problems that cause internal problems. But if most of my patients eat well and avoid poor eating habits, why doesn't their digestive system work well? The answer is that the function of the digestive system must not only be strong enough to process food, but emotions and stress as well. If you cannot process the amount of stress and excess emotions that you deal with on a daily basis, then your digestive system will eventually malfunction. Analyzing my patient data along with data from our Dragon's Way program, I discovered that virtually all of these individuals (several thousand at least) have different degrees of digestive system problems, no matter how well or how little they eat. Food itself is *not* the problem.

So far we've said nothing about calories, fats, sugar, meat, salt, cholesterol, or any of the things you would expect me to talk about in a diet or weight management book. Yet this is a very serious book about weight and healing the root cause of weight problems, so that they do not recur. As you can see, I am going deeper inside your body and talking about the miraculous system that keeps your body, mind, emotions and spirit functioning as one healthy, indivisible system.

A QUICK LOOK AT TYPICAL WEIGHT LOSS PROGRAMS

Generally speaking, there are three types of weight loss programs popular today. One type focuses on diet alone. This kind of program has several variations. Some talk about controlling the quantity or portions of food you eat, or limiting types of foods you eat, and/or controlling the quantity based on any number of nutrient combinations. Another prevalent type of weight loss program is one that promotes the use of herbs, and/or vitamins, and nutritional supplements to suppress your appetite. And the third major program is a combination of one of these two food restriction programs plus a lot of strenuous exercise. Many programs also offer support in the form of weekly meetings or one-on-one counseling sessions, as well as preplanned and prepackaged meals that you can buy. I believe many of these programs can help you lose weight, but they do not help you heal its root cause.

Many of you have probably tried one or more of these weight loss programs and diets. Many of you have probably devised your own form of diet. Given the fact that you're now reading this book, chances are you are among the overwhelming majority of people who have regained at least some or all of the weight you have worked hard to take off. Perhaps, even worse, you have regained more than you had originally lost.

I know that this cycle must be exceedingly frustrating. I can't tell you how many times people come to The Dragon's Way program and say, "I hope this time I can take the weight off for good." Or they tell me, "Maybe I can lose some weight because it is affecting my health and diets aren't working for me anymore." These are intelligent, motivated people who do not understand why the diet programs they went on were unsuccessful. Often they are hard on themselves and take all the blame. That's very common. And to me, this is very sad. I feel badly for these people because they are missing information that could relieve both their physical and emotional distress. In some cases, they have progressed beyond distress to despair. Many people have told me that over and over again in the past they resolved "to be good" this time or "to do it right," then they "cheated," "binged," or just "gave up." They often feel that it's their fault because they weren't able to stick with the other plans. Quitting made them feel guilty and like a failure. For some, this negative cycle has literally changed their personality.

I tell my patients and my Dragon's Way participants that I look at their situation very differently. I think that this inability to stick to a particular plan or diet might have been because they were actually listening to their body's wisdom. It's clear to me that in many of these cases, their body knew the weight loss plan they were on was not healthy for them if they stayed on it for an extended period of time. In other cases, the overwhelming desire for certain "forbidden foods" actually may have been a message from their body of what it really needed, but the message was misinterpreted or misunderstood. People who have gone through The Dragon's Way program understand, at last, that they are not weak-willed or failures, that they are not stupid or ineffectual, that they are not lazy or unmotivated, but rather that they were on programs that simply could not heal the real source of their problem. The following stories of two of our participants might seem familiar to you.

Fatigue, shortness of breath, memory problems, anxiety, poor circulation, and headaches were a regular part of my life much longer than the extra fifteen pounds I wanted to lose. I'm forty-five, but there were days when I felt much older. I had tried a number of different programs over the years. I think I've lost the same ten pounds about six or seven times. Up until recently, I was able to keep my weight relatively stable. Then even though I was working with a trainer, eating a low-fat, low-calorie diet the way I had been taught, I could not get my weight to budge. I always had this vague feeling that some of my health complaints were somehow related to the extra weight, but I had no way to understand how. Everything I heard or read focused on externals such as the food, the calories, the free weights, etc.

   I started The Dragon's Way and added the Wu Ming *Meridian Therapy Qigong immediately a few times a week at first. I must confess that I was more conscientious about applying the principles of Eating for Healing. Then I realized the Qigong practice was strengthening my ability to cope with stress, so I did more. By the end of the program, I no longer felt fatigued and was so much calmer. The shortness of breath disappeared in my fourth week and I no longer have headaches regularly. This program helped me relate to food in a different way. Today my food choices are based more on my body's needs, which I can now tune in to very well.*

I'm someone who does new things slowly. The program was like putting my toe in the water and I then waded in up to my knees by the time it was over. I've learned the TCM principles and understand how to apply them to my life, especially Qigong and eating energy healing foods. I've seen amazing results in my overall health and so I know that this works. The fifteen pounds I took off became a side benefit.

LUCINDA P., 45-YEAR-OLD ADVERTISING VICE PRESIDENT

Here's another perspective:

In the past, I mainly used my own "starvation programs" even though I have some heart problems. I really hated the idea of being overweight. I believed in strictly controlling food intake to control weight, even when it didn't work for me. In the six weeks of The Dragon's Way, my overall health has improved significantly. I've been able to eliminate shortness of breath, fatigue, heavy perspiration, bloating, various menstrual problems and anger that was so chronic I was thinking of seeing a therapist. I took off about twenty-three pounds and approximately ten inches overall. This is not a "quick fix" program. It's one that teaches you how to take care of yourself for life. Eating is a new adventure now because I understand how food can help me heal by giving me the energy or Qi that I need to live well. I particularly enjoyed eating the vegetables. Everything tastes different now. My senses have perked up and I am much calmer at work.

TERRY W., 48-YEAR-OLD PUBLIC ADMINISTRATOR

Sometimes you just have to use common sense about some of these diet programs. Let's take appetite-suppressing plans, for example. Or the kind that limit you to a small amount of calories per day. Appetite-suppressing programs and products and strict portion control plans can only take you so far. Sooner or later, you must stop them because they do not offer you a sustainable, healthy way to live your life. If you had a child and he or she wasn't hungry day after day, wouldn't you be concerned about his or her health? Instinctively you know that this is not a good situation and would start looking for the cause of the poor appetite and seek immediate ways to remedy this problem.

From the TCM perspective, it's not healthy for anyone of any age *not* to be hungry. Being hungry is a signal from your body (not your mind). There's also another, even deeper reason that these appetite suppressants concern me. They send the wrong message to your organs. Here's what they're telling your body: "You can reduce or stop performing your natural functions." In this case, the first organ function that appetite suppressants affect is the liver. Because good health and balanced weight are dependent on the strong and harmonious functioning of all your organs, to upset that balance can potentially cause physical problems. Also, in a practical sense, it makes it even harder for you to maintain your weight loss once you're off the herbs or vitamins, nutritional supplements, or suppressants. In effect, these products can cause your organs to develop a kind of amnesia. When you stop taking them, your organs, especially the liver, first have to "relearn" their true function to become balanced again. Then they have to work very hard and use extra Qi to fix any damage. No wonder excess weight returns. There's no energy capacity left for healing the root problem—everyone's busy fixing up the house!

TCM teaches that when the function of the digestive organs are balanced and a person's Qi is strong, then enormous appetite or wild food cravings are virtually impossible. Ideally, the healthy body only asks for what it actually needs. In TCM, signals of hunger and desires for certain foods are recognized as messages from the body for the delivery of a specific kind of Qi that it needs to function and maintain balance. Unfortunately, in Western society we've conditioned ourselves to "think what we need" rather than to "feel what we need." I urge you to begin to practice this simple exercise that can help recall or reawaken this body memory. Sit quietly before a meal and see if you *feel* hungry, or if you *think* you are hungry. What's the difference? Can you tell? Try to become sensitive to this difference. After a meal, see if you *feel* full or if you *think* you are full. What's the difference? Relying on our minds rather than our feelings as the basis regarding hunger is often the source of unhealthy eating habits. Therefore, an important goal of The Dragon's Way is to heal your digestive system and at the same time increase your awareness of and responsiveness to the messages that your body is sending.

Approaching the solution to weight problems from the vantage point of controlling caloric, fat, fiber, carbohydrate, and/or protein measurements is guaranteed to keep you viewing "food as the enemy." One Dragon's Way graduate expressed her new perspective this way:

> *Prior to The Dragon's Way, I'd have a running dialogue with myself that used to go on about food all the time. "Should I eat this? Will my dress fit if I eat this? Will I be able to go to the gym and work off these calories? Should I make a dinner date this week or will I end up eating too much? Should I eat breakfast today if I am going out to lunch? Maybe I should skip dinner. If I eat a salad for lunch and dinner today, then tomorrow I can eat cake. I can't buy that for my family because I am likely to eat it too. If I have a glass of wine at dinner with my husband, will it keep me from losing weight this week?" I spent more time thinking about how to protect myself from food than anything else. Life was a continual mental*

struggle that revolved around food and dieting and I felt I was always losing. I am so grateful to The Dragon's Way. It finally helped me break out of this constant running dialogue about food and its "bad" effect on my body. Now, I hardly ever even think of food. My responses are natural and healthy. I eat what I want. I have a glass of wine with my husband and really enjoy it without any guilt. And, it's amazing to me how much time I have to think about other things and appreciate the great people and things in my life.

DINA L., 39-YEAR-OLD FASHION CONSULTANT/BUSINESS OWNER

Some diet programs are about food control. Common approaches are to practice portion control, minimize your contact with food, beware of hidden fat or calories, store foods you like in the back of closets and the refrigerator, restrict where you eat, only buy treats for your family that you don't like, and keep a daily record of everything that you eat and drink. One of my students calls this last behavior modification strategy "spying on yourself"! While these strategies may be helpful for a time, and may all sound somewhat reasonable, these kinds of measures do not educate you about how to truly heal and take care of yourself and empower you to listen to what your body needs. Above all, they do not help you learn how to increase Qi so that you can bring your organs into balance and harmony again.

A fairly typical food control program breakfast is one slice of toast, one soft-boiled egg, and half a grapefruit. On some days this can be quite filling, on other days, it is not. So you may guiltily eat the other half of grapefruit. Because you are operating out of guilt, perhaps the next day you'll have two slices of toast until finally, ten days later, you're no longer on the diet. Again, food becomes something it shouldn't: a thing with which you struggle.

WHY THE DRAGON'S WAY IS DIFFERENT

The Dragon's Way uses a three-pronged formula that has been carefully designed to address the root cause of excess weight conditions. It lets you increase and improve the function of your Qi, so that you can recall your own healing ability and bring your body back into balance. When this happens, you *can* lose weight, and just as important, you will be energized and healed in ways that you might never have imagined! I think you can now begin to understand that this is not what most Westerners think of as a "diet."

The Dragon's Way is a self-healing program based on centuries of success. It is a six-week journey, after a week of preparation. Over the course of these six weeks, the average participant takes off about twelve pounds and eight inches overall from her or his body. Some take off more; others less. However, in addition to the weight and inches, people also find that their eating patterns and food likes and dislikes evolve. Others discover that they have been able to heal or greatly reduce their fatigue, insomnia, digestive disturbances, nervousness, worrying, depression, anger, and/or headaches. Additionally, many experience dramatic improvements in their cholesterol levels, hypertension, hot flashes, and PMS symptoms. Some have had other unexpected results, such as the one participant who found that foot pain, which had plagued her for several decades, gradually vanished as she began to strengthen her body's Qi reserves.

Here's what she told us:

When I started this program, I was very focused on losing weight. I never thought it would help me with my feet! I had so many problems with my feet. I was especially bothered by pain on the bottom of my feet and toes. It never occurred to me that my foot pain was affecting other parts of me. I had been to many, many Western doctors. No one was able to help me or tell me what was wrong, so I gave away practically all of my beautiful shoes because almost all of them

hurt my feet. I wish I could get my shoes back because I no longer have any pain!
CHERYL R., 41-YEAR-OLD SYSTEMS ANALYST

You might think that it's very unusual for foot pain to be alleviated through a program that address weight problems. But as we discussed, this is not an ordinary program. This woman's long-time foot pain was related to her kidney and bladder. The meridians of both of these organs begin or end in the foot, and both organs were out of balance and not functioning in harmony or "speaking" to each other. Practicing two of The Dragon's Way movements, *The Dragon Kicks Backward* (#8) and *The Dragon Stands Between Heaven and Earth* (#10), helped strengthen the function of these two organs and helped Qi flow more smoothly through their meridians. When this happened, her foot pain healed.

Another participant said:

My job as an expediter in a busy company is high stress. I didn't take The Dragon's Way because I needed to lose weight but because I had so many stress-related physical and emotional symptoms that my friend who took the program thought I really needed help and recommended it. I gave it a try because I am too young to feel this bad. I'm thirty-eight years old and before I took The Dragon's Way I was tired all the time, had shortness of breath, back pain, muscle tension, depression, anxiety, poor circulation, and heart palpitations. What bothered me most of all were these really awful nightmares. Week after week these incredible nightmares were ruining my sleep. I had to do something. I'm relieved to say, my friend was right. I learned how to use TCM self-healing knowledge to bring my body back into balance. In just six weeks, I no longer experienced any of the above symptoms. I am still amazed by how good I feel! Best of all, those awful nightmares are gone. I have reclaimed a good night's sleep for myself.
MARK V., 38-YEAR-OLD EXPEDITER, IMPORT/EXPORT BUSINESS

TCM understands that nightmares are usually related to an imbalance in the relationship between the heart and the kidney. Sometimes, nightmares can be the result of a function disorder of the liver and its partner organ the gallbladder. In this case, Qigong directly helped this participant restore balance between his organs and the nightmares disappeared.

As you go through this book and our Dragon's Way program, it is my job to help you understand at a deep level that everyone is born with the gift to self-heal. Perhaps you are already aware of this innate ability. Think about it. When you have a cold or the flu, you recover. When you pull a muscle, it gets better. When you have a headache, it eventually goes away. How do you suppose all this happens? It happens because your body has a myriad of healing mechanisms. It has its own tool kit of various chemical and even natural antibiotics and drugs. You may think it's the aspirin or Tylenol that's gotten rid of your headache, but in reality, these substances have just suppressed your headache's symptoms so that your own healing mechanisms could help your body rebalance itself.

The healing abilities of our bodies are remarkable. They can heal far more complicated problems than headaches, especially with the help of a self-healing practice like the Qigong you will work with in The Dragon's Way. With the proper knowledge and practice, everyone can tap into this remarkable healing ability and become balanced. When we do, one of the results is taking off excess weight and inches. That is what The Dragon's Way is all about.

EXCESS WEIGHT: IS THERE A REAL VILLAIN?

In my healing practice, my work is not directed solely at treating the condition (no matter what it is) that my patients walk in with. My true work is aimed at helping them learn how they became unbalanced or unwell in the first place and what the root cause of their health problems is. Once they understand this, I teach them how to take care of their body, mind, emotions, and spirit, so that they do not become sick again. TCM's real specialty is prevention. I do not want to see you when you are sick. I want to see you when you are well so that we can both work on minor things and keep you from falling out of balance in the first place. It might interest you to know that in ancient China, the TCM practitioner did not get paid if his or her patient became ill. Why? Quite simply because the doctor had not done his job of keeping his patient well! It's the same when I work with people who are dealing with weight issues. I want you to learn how to heal the root cause so you can prevent this problem from recurring in your life and making you miserable.

So what are the root causes of excess weight? I have been told that every successful "diet" book must have a villain. Over the years, dieters have had a huge variety of books with a long list of "bad guys" from which to choose. There are calories, carbohydrates, fats, sugar, cholesterol, meat, dairy. Then, of course, there's overeating, not getting enough exercise, and not consuming the "right" foods in the "right" combinations, and even bad thoughts or not enough prayer!

I have interesting news for you. From the TCM perspective, the real villain is none of the above. It's chronic, unrelenting stress. I like to make a joke with my patients. I tell them: "Stress . . . made in the USA!" You may be skeptical at first, but as you read on, you will learn how stress unbalances the function of one of your most important organs, and how that affects the other organs with which it has relationships. Inside our bodies, everything is connected. You cannot damage one thing without affecting others. I urge you to think about this. While Western medicine focuses on treating the disease, TCM's interest lies in treating the whole person.

When I first came to the United States, I was struck by the number of overweight people. I was really surprised at the statistics as well, but when I started my practice in TCM, I began to understand what was going on. Immediately, I could see that the stress, worry, and even fear, that many people live with was undermining and unbalancing the way the body is designed to work. Stress is the number one external factor creating this unhealthful situation. And it doesn't seem that stress is going away any time soon. A recent study by the International Labor Organization cited that the number of hours Americans work has increased dramatically. Americans have now taken first place in the working hours lottery with 1,966 hours each year, surpassing even the hardworking Japanese by about 70 hours. And we work 350 more hours, or nine more weeks, than Europeans. Discussing the study in a recent *New York Times* article, Harvard professor Juliet Schor commented, "A very significant group, roughly a third of the labor force, is working more hours than they want. They are feeling high levels of time pressure and stress. They feel their job interferes with their family life." She noted that stress is being experienced in particular by baby boomers.

I believe the more stressed out people become, the more weight problems we will see. In fact, I think weight problems will reach almost epidemic proportions. We can add to this a kind of hypnosis that is pushed on us by media of all kinds. Every major magazine, even health magazines, show us images that are supposed to represent vibrant, healthy, happy individuals. Television does not offer us much better. These images, of course, aren't real, but we all basically receive the same message: "If you don't look like this, you are not healthy." This isn't true. Every one of us is a unique and beautiful energy being. We can all reach a state of optimum health, but unfortunately, we will probably never see this reflected in the contemporary media.

Pinning weight problems on stress may seem like a simplistic explanation until you understand this concept from the TCM perspective. It's important to understand that stress is not something you experience in your mind: you feel it in every part of your body, and it has an effect on every body structure. In this program, you will begin to understand how stress dives deep into the body to disrupt relationships among the organs and create havoc with their healthy functioning. One of the results is your organs can no longer perform all the jobs they're supposed to do, including helping you to automatically remain at your best weight.

In The Dragon's Way, we continually educate our participants about how important it is to understand that stress takes its toll both externally and internally. All of us are so continually bombarded with stress and stressful situations that many people do not recognize the debilitating role stress plays in their lives. They live with high levels of stress because they think "that's just the way things are." But that's not the way things need to be, especially if you want to solve weight problems at their core. I don't have to tell you that stress is our constant companion and that people who are plagued with obvious stress-related problems such as tension headaches, stomachaches, and neck pain know too well how it can rob their lives of fun and a feeling of well-being.

TCM recognizes that stress is particularly hard on your liver. When this important organ starts to malfunction, it communicates its unhappiness to all the other major organs—liver, heart, spleen and stomach, lung, and kidney. Like a shock wave spreading out through your body, its vibrations begin to destabilize the functions of your other organs.

As a small business owner, my life is incredibly busy and filled with stress. Having two small children is wonderful, but they also demand a lot of energy and sometimes this creates more stress. Of course, I never really connected stress with my weight problems until I met Dr. Lu and began The Dragon's Way. I had used a variety of diet programs and products, not to mention really intense workouts at the gym

over the years to take off weight. The truth is I never experi-
enced anything like this. I practiced Qigong almost every day
and the change in my energy is incredible! My nervousness
disappeared along with my stomach bloat and the headaches
that started like clockwork every day around 3:00 P.M. This
is a program for life. The more I apply it, the better it gets.
I never expected to lose twenty-five pounds in six weeks! For
me this program has just begun.

VINNIE G., 38-YEAR-OLD COMPUTER STORE OWNER

Our bodies are like miracle workers. Given the intensity with which we live our modern lifestyle, our bodies are always working to become balanced so that we can remain in good health. But it requires Qi to accomplish this task. If our Qi reserves are low and internal organs are compromised or not functioning well, we cannot fight off the things that are bombarding us. The result: illness, disease, and for some people, the frustrating condition of excess weight or stubborn weight retention.

With The Dragon's Way, I have taken the best of TCM's ancient principles to create a program that really works for today's men and women—men and women whose lives are like nonstop roller coasters. Although the specific requirements of The Dragon's Way are few, if you give them your full attention and commitment, I believe you will achieve some amazing results. Remember, you will not find any other program like this.

UNDERSTANDING THE ESSENCE OF THE DRAGON'S WAY

I hope by now that you'd like to explore The Dragon's Way more deeply and learn how it differs from other programs you've tried. You are about to embark on a serious healing program based on ancient TCM principles. While it only lasts six weeks after an initial preparation week, my wish for you is that it lasts a lifetime!

The Dragon's Way uses a unique combination of three very powerful self-healing tools. They are:

- Practicing ten simple "energy movements" called *Wu Ming* Meridian Therapy Qigong.
- Following a specially designed "Eating for Healing" plan to strengthen and increase your Qi.
- Learning how your body really works from the TCM perspective.

When we conduct The Dragon's Way in person, there are two other components that are included to help give participants the best chance of healing. These items can help enhance your experience with The Dragon's Way; however, it's important to note that without them you should obtain excellent results if you follow the program as it's outlined here. These are:

- Two herbal supplements: *Imperial Qi* and *Green Dragon*. Each is adapted exclusively for Western individuals from an ancient, natural formula that has been in use for centuries. These are not appetite suppressants. They are herbs that go to specific organs associated with weight management problems and help rebalance their function as well as encourage harmony between the organs. Remember, we are always working at getting your own healing ability to "kick in" and take over this process. If you want to boost your healing program, you can order these herbs from our Foundation. The address can be found at the back of this book. These two formulas have been in use since the beginning of The Dragon's Way and many, many participants have had excellent results with them.
- The Dragon's Way Audiotape: We have developed this special audiocassette to help encourage participants in their daily practice. Against a background of my special "music for

healing," participants can listen to the count on each of the Qigong movements and practice with me in real time. The second side features a full thirty-minute meditation of Taoist energy music. Again, this audiotape can be ordered from our Foundation.

Opening a Secret Door to Healing with Qigong

The Dragon's Way can work for you if you work with all three of the essential components. They are meant to work together as a powerful healing system that will help you give up twelve pounds or more and eight inches within the six-week program period. Why do I say "give up"? It's a different concept than "losing." What happens when you lose something? You try to find it and get it back. I want you to change your concept about weight entirely. I don't want you to lose it; I want you to give it up or give it away (maybe you have some thin friends who could use some extra weight?). Your thoughts are powerful, and it is important to help yourself think within a totally different frame of reference.

The cornerstone of The Dragon's Way is the *Wu Ming* Meridian Therapy Qigong movements. Qigong is an ancient energy practice that has been used by the Chinese throughout the ages as a way to help the body, mind, and spirit work as one holistic system. The specific Qigong movements that I've chosen are from a tradition known as *Wu Ming* Qigong. Here, we are going to apply them as meridian therapy to accomplish two things: to help your body's organ systems work in harmony and to relieve the blockages of Qi that are the root cause of excess weight. Like a jumpstart, these Qigong movements can help your Qi flow smoothly throughout your body. A good TCM doctor knows that by increasing and strengthening the flow of a person's Qi, everything inside the body can change. Things such as mucus and water and fat get stuck in our bodies. By getting your internal battery functioning again and getting Qi to flow, the whole body gets better *evenly*. That's why fat and water are eliminated naturally and muscles can become more toned—even without strenuous exercises.

Our Dragon's Way *Wu Ming* Meridian Therapy Qigong movements are gentle and relaxing. They are not physical exercises intended to develop muscles. You may, however, find that you're more flexible after practicing these movements because they gently stretch your tendons as well as your meridians. These meridian stretches are designed to help relieve hunger, stimulate your own healing ability, and increase Qi. To work successfully with The Dragon's Way, it is very important to practice these movements daily. They take only about twenty minutes to do from start to finish. Practicing these movements after you complete the six-week program of The Dragon's Way will help you to continue your journey to greater health and to maintain the benefits you achieved during the program.

Eating for a Greater Purpose: Healing

During the course of The Dragon's Way, you will learn about food from a completely different perspective. First of all, food will no longer be your enemy. Rather, it will become your friend and your partner.

TCM values food as a source of healing and Qi. TCM states that each food has its own signature Qi or essence and at least one healing purpose. Thus, I have chosen each food specifically for its healing ability and for its role in helping your body pass out water and eliminate body fat. My goal is to enable your body to experience a cleanup and tuneup at its deepest level. Consequently, I've selected foods that not only will help heal specific organs, but also will be gentle on your body and do not demand a great deal of Qi or energy to digest. I also ask that you eat so you are 70 percent full. If you eat a little less, you will need less Qi to digest your food. This helps you conserve Qi and apply your reserve to the healing process. When you do this, the weight comes off.

You will see that eating becomes a different experience because you are not eating to survive, but eating for healing. When food is consumed in this way, it gives the body energy in accordance with its current need. When you learn to listen to your body's requests and honor those messages, you automatically give yourself the correct balance of healing foods for your health and lifestyle.

As you embark on this journey, I want to emphasize once again that The Dragon's Way is not a diet! It's really a gateway that you can open to a whole new life.

Learning to Look at Your Body and Your Health the TCM Way

I've structured this book to reflect the way we conduct The Dragon's Way Program. The participants meet once a week. The first twenty minutes is spent doing the *Wu Ming* Meridian Therapy Qigong movements together. It's very helpful and powerful to practice with other people. Why? Because with each additional person, the energy field can be amplified or magnified, and this adds more power to the healing process. If you can encourage a few people to participate in The Dragon's Way with you, try doing the exercises together and you'll see what I mean.

After we've finished the Qigong movements, I spend the next forty minutes or so of the class giving what I call a lesson about TCM. I talk about many things, but it is essential that our Dragon's Way participants learn about the key TCM theories: Qi and Blood, Meridian and Organ Systems, the Theory of Yin/Yang, and The Five Element Theory.

Beginning in Week 2, I then talk each week about one of the body's five main organs—liver, heart, spleen, lung, and kidney—their individual Qi, and their relationships with one another. In Part II, I do the same thing at the end of each weekly session. You'll find that this book contains a great deal of interesting ancient healing wisdom. While I did not create this information, it is my mission and my privilege to bring this time-tested knowledge to as many people as possible, especially in the West. Because some of this information runs counter to prevailing Western thinking, I urge you to read and reread each chapter so you can gain a deeper appreciation of these healing concepts that have been continuously and successfully practiced for thousands of years.

Making The Dragon's Way Your Way

For some reason (the ancient Chinese would call it fate), I have received special knowledge—or what is called the keys to special understanding—from my masters that can really help Western men and women with the challenges of modern day life. I am honored to help educate you on how to regain your health, rebalance your body, and prevent illness or disease.

The Chinese like to say: "You eat for someone else's stomach." Why? Because many people, especially in Western cultures where the food is plentiful, interesting, and delicious, select items that make their mouths feel good, but are, in the long term, damaging to the healthy functioning of their major organs, especially their stomach.

As you will see throughout this book, the concept of "eating for healing" goes much deeper than the scientific aspect of foods like calories, nutritional properties, vitamins, and the like. It gets at the very essence of certain foods and which organs they can help heal. In my opinion, it is essential that everyone learn how to eat for health, healing, and building Qi. This is one daily activity where you have maximum control over making positive contributions to your health. Approached properly, this is one powerful way to prevent illness and disease that is often underestimated in the West.

Even though I've been privileged to work with many masters who, in turn, have revealed and passed to me tremendous secret healing skills for pain and injury (especially sports injury), and even though I have practiced the martial arts for thirty-six years, it seems that the Universe has other things in mind for me. It has charged me with the mission of working with men and women in the Western culture so that I can share what I have learned and what I know.

Part of my job is to help you understand that your thoughts are far more powerful and have far more energy than your actions. In my role as a healer, I must help my patients learn how to transform fear, worry, anxiety, anger, and stress into powerful healing tools. I would also like to do that for you. Hope, peacefulness, and confidence in your own healing ability (which, by the way, you were born with) can help you make profound changes in your life.

SOME SUGGESTIONS BEFORE YOU BEGIN

Before you begin The Dragon's Way, I would like to make a few suggestions that I think will help to make the experience easier and more enjoyable for you.

First of all, try not to read this entire book all at once. Rather, start each of the six weeks by reading the chapter specifically for that week. In other words, do the program as if you were actually attending a class that week. Everything you need to complete The Dragon's Way successfully is here. Be sure to review TCM: Self-Healing Tools for Life in the following section before you begin.

In the preparation week before beginning The Dragon's Way, gradually eliminate meat, fowl, fish, and cheese from your meals. This will prepare your body for the upcoming weeks of the program. Why do I recommend doing this? The answer is not what you think. It is not because of the physical properties of these particular foods. I am looking at them from the TCM perspective. Most of them put too much of a burden on your body to digest them. This is Qi you can start to conserve immediately for the more important purpose of self-healing! Remember, everything that we will do over the next six weeks has a healing purpose. The goal is to increase your body's own Qi so that it will cause your organs to function in harmony again. When you reach this state, your weight will begin to drop off naturally and automatically. In other words, your self-regulating capacity will have come back online. After this, you should be able to eat what you want in moderation. However, if you've followed the program properly, what you want may surprise you!

I always tell my Dragon's Way participants to eat their favorite meal and have their favorite dessert or snack sometime before beginning the first week of the program. I suggest you do the same as well. Why? You may think it's because the program intends to "take them away from you" or because they are "forbidden." Once again, the answer is probably not what you think. I recommend this as a kind of *"bon voyage party"* for your taste buds. Believe it or not, some people find that after they complete The Dragon's Way, they're no longer interested in the foods that they once loved—foods that they couldn't see living without—their most favorite foods!

Some people tell me with a mixture of sadness and relief that they just can't get the same feeling again from eating their favorite box of cookies, or that pint of full-fat ice cream, or the sixteen-ounce steak that used to make their mouth water. They are shocked at their indifference to these things. They've developed a new skill, a skill that you can develop if you follow this program and practice *Wu Ming* Meridian Therapy Qigong movements daily. Now, they want to eat fresh foods. Some participants can even tell me which of their local supermarkets have the freshest produce. Why? Because their bodies have recovered the ability to tell fresh, healthy food from stale, underripe or overripe fruits and vegetables. Soon, you too will be able to listen to your body.

Working as a registered nurse, I thought I understood and practiced healthy eating. What I couldn't understand was why I couldn't lose the weight I had put on slowly over the years, and why I couldn't maintain the pounds I managed to lose from dieting and exercise. I "gave up" fourteen pounds and eight inches over the course of this program. I wasn't even thinking about weight loss after the first week. I was concentrating on how much I was learning. This program gave me an entirely new way of understanding what it means to eat for health and healing and how to really enjoy living. I practiced the Qigong movements every day and added the recommended energy healing foods into my diet so that they were mainly what I ate. I don't even need to look at food lists any more. Through The Dragon's Way I learned to really listen to my body and now it actually tells me what it wants. Fruits and vegetables have taken on a whole new perspective in my life. I feel so energized and happy.

MEREDITH J., 54-YEAR-OLD REGISTERED NURSE

When you finish Week 1 in Chapter 5, you will fill out a TCM self-healing checklist. Later on, I'll ask you to fill out a different checklist. These lists will help you evaluate your experience with The Dragon's Way and let you see the progress that you've made in a variety of areas, especially the loss of weight and inches. What you may notice first is that health conditions, such as migraines or headaches, stomach distention, constipation, and more, have positive changes during these weeks. Look at these changes as signs that your body is truly beginning to heal the root cause of your imbalances. You're beginning to look at life The Dragon's Way.

PART I

TCM: SELF-HEALING TOOLS FOR LIFE

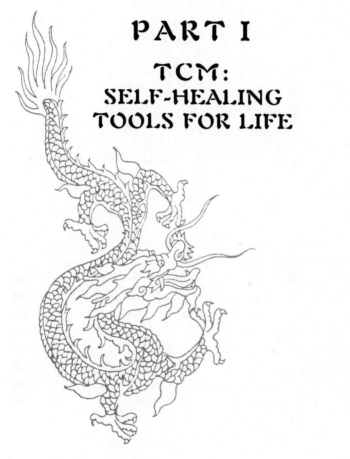

CHAPTER 2
FOODS THAT HEAL:
The Dragon's Way Eating for Healing Plan

INEVITABLY, those who participate in our program want to know, "What can I eat?" Before we list the food selection, I'd like to introduce you to the TCM perspective on how and why certain foods heal the body and increase your all-important Qi. I have chosen each of the foods listed for their healing properties, which go beyond their physical ones.

For many centuries, TCM practitioners have passed down their knowledge of the healing property of foods. This aspect goes beyond calories, nutrition, phytonutrients, vitamins, minerals, and other scientific or physical properties. Again, it has to do with the very real, yet intangible aspect, of Qi or healing essence of a particular food. To follow are the foods that heal that I have chosen for The Dragon's Way. These foods specifically address the organs related to weight problems: the liver, kidney, spleen, and lung. Later in the book, we will go into greater detail about how foods can heal. At this point, it's important to know that the healing energies or essences of these specific foods will actually travel to a specific organ to help strengthen it and help it rebalance and heal itself. As the organ heals, its ability to communicate with other organs is improved as well. These foods can also help your body cleanse itself and your palate so it will be better able later to tell you what is good, fresh, and nourishing.

These foods can be eaten in any combination. I suggest you follow our recommendations for quantities, but The Dragon's Way is not about counting calories, or giving up everything you like. If you feel you need to eat more, then go ahead. This program is about making you feel well and happy, not sad and deprived.

Here is the complete list of recommended foods for The Dragon's Way.

FOODS FOR HEALING THE ROOT CAUSE OF EXCESS WEIGHT AND INCREASING QI

Fruits
Kiwis
Mangos
Oranges
Papaya
Pears
Persimmons
Red apples (Gala, Macintosh, Washington State)
Red grapefruit
Red grapes (about 1 cup)
Strawberries (about 1 cup)
Tangerines
Watermelon (about 1 cup)
(*Note:* There is a healing purpose to choosing red fruits, which I will explain later.)

Vegetables
Baby corn
Bamboo shoots

Bean curd
Broccoli
Broccoli rabe
Carrots
Cauliflower
Celery
Chicory
Eggplant
Fennel
Green pepper
Lotus
Mushrooms
Parsley
Plum tomatoes
Scallions
Seaweed (all kinds)
Water chestnuts
Yellow squash
Zucchini

Nuts/Spices/Oils
Black and white pepper
Black and white sesame seeds
Cashews
Chestnuts
Chili pepper
Cinnamon
Cloves
Garlic
Ginger
Lotus seed
Mint
Olive oil
Pine nuts
Safflower oil

Salt
Sesame oil
Soy sauce
Walnut oil
Walnuts

Others

Bee pollen
Coffee
Egg whites, cooked
Honey
Pasta (any kind)
Rice (any kind)
Tea (preferably Chinese herbal tea)

RECOMMENDED MEALS

Suggested Breakfast

Toasted walnuts (10 halves) and one of the following:
(a) one glass of watermelon juice (including some of the white and green parts of the rind). You can make watermelon juice with a juicer or in a blender. For a blender, you will need to cut up the rind into smaller parts.
(b) apple juice
(c) orange juice
(d) one piece or serving of recommended fruit

Lunch

Two pieces or servings of recommended fruit. For red grapes and strawberries, eat a cup of fruit or more if you feel hungry. In the beginning, before you build up your Qi reserves with *Wu Ming* Meridian Therapy, you may need a little extra food in the morning. You can add more roasted walnuts and more fruit if you like.

If you feel you are hungry (not think you are), there is a special breathing exercise that you can do to alleviate this feeling. These people learned a lot about managing hunger.

Here's what they said:

I really liked the Wu Ming *Meridian Therapy and did it every day with my husband. This was the best nonexercise I ever did! I felt relaxed and energized afterwards and it made my day less stressful. I understand now how the body can self-heal when it becomes balanced and how to apply the various parts of the program to my life. I can hardly believe that I lost thirty pounds in six weeks and ate and only experienced a little hunger at the beginning of the program. I know it was strengthening my Qi that made me progressively less hungry as the program went on.*

LINDA T., 43-YEAR-OLD HOUSEWIFE, MOTHER OF TWO

This program changed my weight and my understanding about health. I took off fifteen pounds and six inches. The meridian stretches are a wonderful way to start the day. I think that doing them every morning is what has helped me to feel clearer and more calm. I followed the Eating for Healing plan from the very beginning as a challenge and I was never hungry. I thought that maybe I would be hungry throughout the day, but I was very full all of the time. This surprised me because I had been on traditional diet programs that used a lot of the same foods, but naturally none was dealing with the root cause of my weight problem. Nor were any of them able to strengthen my Qi. I really like the change in how I think about food. This is much simpler than counting calories or fat. I am much more aware of what my body really needs and how to get it.

CINDY F., 42-YEAR-OLD TECHNICAL WRITER

Dinner

Two or three portions of recommended vegetables. Try to eat a variety of recommended vegetables at each meal. See if you can prepare three different-colored vegetables. Each color belongs to and can help heal a specific organ in The Five Element Theory. For example, baby corn is yellow and is good for your stomach and spleen; celery is green and is good for your liver; fennel is white and is good for your lung and kidney. These vegetables may be steamed, sautéed, stir-fried, braised, roasted, grilled, or prepared as soup. Do not fry, deep fry, or barbecue. Eat more if you feel hungry. You can also add a half-cup of any kind of rice or pasta.

Snack: Eat more fruit, or have a cup of tea with walnuts or pine nuts.

TCM TIP TO INCREASE QI AND ELIMINATE HUNGER

This special five-minute meditation can be done anytime and anywhere. It can relax your mind, increase your Qi, and help eliminate feelings of hunger. I recommend that you include it in your daily routine whenever you feel hungry.

Reverse Breathing

Stand or sit in any position that makes you comfortable. Close your eyes and slowly breathe in with your nose. While you breathe in, pull your stomach in. Slowly breathe out from your mouth. When you breathe out, push your stomach out. Count each breath in and out as one. After four or five breaths, breathe in slowly and deeply and hold your breath. Count to five as slowly as you can. Then exhale slowly. Do another set or two of these reverse breathing exercises. They should help you manage any hunger feelings.

Now, after learning about these food recommendations, if we were in class, you would probably ask all kinds of questions, like: Which kind of rice is better, brown or white? Can I eat more than a half-cup of pasta? Is there enough nutrition in your "diet"? I'll be really tired if I don't eat meat! Where's the protein? Can I eat more than one snack? What about coffee, or tea? Should I use low-fat milk or skim milk? Can I use artificial sweeteners? Is it all right to drink wine on The Dragon's Way? And much, much more! We've answered so many of these questions so many times that I thought it would be helpful to create a chapter of those most frequently asked questions. Please turn to Chapter 13 if you'd like to explore this aspect of The Dragon's Way now.

The avalanche of questions comes from so much exposure to Western diets, the Western way of thinking about food, as well as advertising and the numerous articles about weight and weight loss. (This is, after all, a $30-billion-a-year industry.) At first, you may find it almost hard to believe that these simple, everyday foods can help you heal your body. Another reason for so many questions is that participants are conditioned to believe that "eating less" is the reason for any weight loss. This is not the true power of our program. The real difference is *Wu Ming* Meridian Therapy. Healing foods and herbs are secondary. The real proof is when you start to increase Qi and you begin to take off pounds and inches. That's when the magic of this program becomes self-evident. And again, I'd like to emphasize that you are receiving healing knowledge and information that no other weight loss or diet program or product can deliver.

SOME GUIDELINES

If you're used to dieting the American way, the following guidelines may seem a little unusual to you. Each relates to TCM principles that have been practiced for thousands of years; I have not made these things up. These guidelines have been firmly in place in TCM medical texts for a very long time. As you go through each week's lesson on TCM, you will gain a greater understanding (and, I hope, appreciation) for these guidelines and how they underpin all your new healing tools. By the time you finish The Dragon's Way, I promise you will understand why following these guidelines can help you heal and how they contribute to true health.

- Avoid drinking cold fluids.
- If you are used to drinking a lot of water, please stop!
- Only drink room temperature water (never ice water) when you are thirsty.
- Eat only cooked vegetables.
- Avoid fried and barbecued foods.
- Eat only roasted or toasted walnuts, pine nuts, and cashews.
- Eat your heaviest foods only in the morning or early afternoon.
- Eat fruits for lunch and vegetables for dinner.
- Given the complexity of the digestive process, try to eat dinner before 7:00 or 8:00 P.M.
- Eat other fruits and vegetables, but try to stick to the list because they provide a greater healing benefit for weight loss.
- Digestion is a function of the whole body. It applies to food, as well as emotions and spiritual aspects of the soul. Try to process everything you put into your body in a calm, peaceful way.

The following TCM Taste Record provides a way to understand more about how your body speaks to you about the need for certain foods. You can use it during the program to keep track of any specific food cravings, the time of day that they occur, your feelings or emotions at that time. Refer to The Five Element Theory chart on page 133 and fill in the organ that relates to this taste. Food cravings are your body's way of getting attention and letting you know that a specific organ is out of balance. These are not something about which you need to feel guilty, especially if you are a woman and this happens before or during your menstrual cycle. You should be happy that this function is working. Practice listening to your body and not your mind. Keep eating the foods on the recommended list, practice Qigong, and avoid stress. Your food cravings should eventually disappear as your organs become more balanced and your body begins to work in harmony.

TCM TASTE RECORD

Time of day: _____

Taste desired: _____

My feelings: _____

_____

_____

I have been thinking about: _____

_____

_____

Organ that relates to this taste: _____

Time of day: _____

Taste desired: _____

My feelings: _____

_____

_____

I have been thinking about: _____

_____

_____

Organ that relates to this taste: _____

Time of day: _____

Taste desired: _____

My feelings: _____

_____

_____

I have been thinking about: _____

_____

_____

Organ that relates to this taste: _____

Time of day: _____

Taste desired: _____

My feelings: _____

_____

_____

I have been thinking about: _____

_____

_____

Organ that relates to this taste: _____

CHAPTER 3

WU MING MERIDIAN THERAPY:
Healing The Dragon's Way with Ancient Qigong Movements That Rebalance Your Body

O_{NE} of my goals in The Dragon's Way is to help educate you as much as I can about how and why this program is unique and what makes it work. The most important part of The Dragon's Way is *Wu Ming* Meridian Therapy. It is ancient healing wisdom that is not available from any other source. I would like to take some time here to educate you a bit deeper about Qigong and its power.

Qigong can do what no other medicine can: help your body, mind, and spirit to connect and function in harmony. It reawakens and strengthens your body's innate healing ability, and lets you tap into the healing energy of the Universe. Qigong has the ability to address the root cause of weight problems. How? Excess weight is the end result or symptom of a chain of internal events that originate with a Qi deficiency and Qi imbalance. This condition then causes several organs to develop a function disorder. This means that these organs cannot perform the tasks that they are programmed to do, such as rid your body of water and fat, regulate your metabolism, protect your immune system, etc. Generally speaking, physical problems such as chronic headaches, allergies of all kinds, asthma, thyroid problems, depression, emotional problems, diabetes, heart disease, and more occur before there is a weight gain. Treating a Qi function disorder is essential to solving weight control issues. Qigong is the best medicine; it is also the most difficult and the most dangerous.

Now, let's explore Qigong, the true foundation of all the Chinese arts: the fine arts, the martial arts, and TCM. All of the famous TCM doctors were also high-level Qigong masters. There are many Qigong systems, based on a variety of principles, but essentially Qigong is learned in two ways: by *forms*, or by *message*. In a Qigong system based on *forms* or *techniques*, you learn a variety of exercises, and the emphasis is on doing these exercises correctly. If you do them right, you can increase your Qi; if not, you won't get the benefit. In a *message* system, you may also learn certain forms, but the essence of the practice is that the message is transferred to you by the master. If you do the forms wrong, you'll still get the benefit. If you are learning by technique, your exercises should be perfect. If you are learning by message, your heart must be empty and open. The Dragon's Way Qigong is one where the message is passed by me in my role as a Qigong master to you.

It is difficult to say how old the practice of Qigong is. Some believe it goes back far more than five thousand years. The word Qigong literally means "energy work," but the actual practice is far deeper than its description. It is a powerful self-healing discipline that is particularly effective for many conditions and is especially good for women who want to prevent or alleviate menopausal symptoms. As we've said, Qigong can help you connect your body, mind, and spirit by allowing you to gain control of and direct your own Qi or life force. Its biggest benefit is that it can develop your intuition and let you see the world in a different way. This view is one that can take you beyond the senses.

There are five distinct Qigong traditions: Taoist, Confucian, Buddhist, martial arts, and medical. It is this last form of Qigong that is beginning to attract a great deal of attention from Western audiences. I say beginning because Qigong was suppressed during the Chinese Cultural Revolution, which roughly lasted from 1965 to 1976. Qigong never died out in practice; around 1978, it began its rise in popularity again in China. More and more people around the world are becoming interested in this ancient energy practice. In 1988, the Chinese held the first World Conference for showcasing Qigong medical research. These conferences have grown over the past decade and have been held in Tokyo, and Berkeley, California.

Qigong is one of the most powerful prescriptions a TCM doctor can use because it works directly on the body's energy system. Today in China, more than 100 million people practice this self-healing energy system daily. Qigong is an ideal prescription for some of my patients and their particular problems. I often teach my patients one or two simple Qigong movements to help them reawaken their healing ability and to speed up their healing process. This is good for them because they now have something to use to heal themselves should they develop the same problem again.

Qigong is particularly good for healing problems that Western medicine cannot identify; frequently these are organ function problems that do not show up on scientific tests. Qigong is very good for helping correct immune system disorders and chronic conditions of many kinds.

In China, medical practitioners have found Qigong effective in treating a wide variety of health conditions, including drug abuse and obesity. In hospitals and clinics across China, Qigong is routinely prescribed to treat arthritis, asthma, bowel problems, diabetes, migraines, hypertension, rheumatism, neuralgia, stress, ulcers, and many other conditions. Qigong has also been used to successfully treat cancers and reduce or even eliminate debilitating side effects of radiation and chemotherapy. It is not uncommon in China for women to recover from breast cancer by practicing Qigong.

It also can bring special relief to those suffering from chronic pain and other chronic conditions that affect the digestive, respiratory, nervous, and cardiovascular systems. Qigong practice has been documented to speed recovery from surgery and sports and other kinds of injuries. I have had great success with prescribing Qigong for a number of patients to help them recover more rapidly from devastating injuries, such as those resulting from car accidents.

Some of the amazing things that Qigong can do are strengthen the immune system, lower blood pressure, adjust pulse rates, help alter metabolic rates, adjust oxygen demand, harmonize endocrine system functions, regulate some of the body's basic building blocks, and even slow the process of aging. Above all, the Qigong practitioner learns through his or her own experience that there is no separation between the body and the mind.

Qigong should not be confused with pure physical exercise. Many studies have been done on Qigong and it is generally acknowledged that in addition to its powers of integration, it offers the benefits of aerobics, meditation, and more.

Thousands of Qigong systems derived from the five basic traditions mentioned above exist in China. Some are ancient systems passed along for many generations; some are "instant systems" created by modern masters. Currently, very few Qigong systems have been seen or taught in the United States. In my Center's school in New York, I teach Taoist *Wu Ming* Qigong, which traces its lineage directly back to the ancient masters *Lao Tzu* (sixth century B.C.) and *Chuang Tzu* (fourth century B.C.).

Each Qigong system works differently: some are easy to learn, but deliver few benefits; some are difficult to learn and the benefits are difficult to achieve; some are difficult to learn, but yield great benefits. I believe the best Qigong system should be easy to learn and should allow you to achieve great benefits. *Wu Ming* Meridian Therapy Qigong is the last kind.

Let's look a little deeper at the two types of Qigong mentioned above: *form* or technique and *message*. Systems in the first category are based on postures and movements that stimulate your internal Qi to help heal yourself. In this case, the practitioner must follow the master's directions precisely to gain any benefits from the system. Results depend on correct posture, how much time you practice, and how well your master can teach. In this system, the connection to posture and getting it correct is more important than the relationship between student and master. With this type of system, the benefits are in proportion to the amount of personal effort you put into the practice.

The second category uses movements and postures, but in a different way. They are used to guide the power of the "energy message" from master to student. Doing the forms or postures correctly is not overly important—they are merely the "the vehicle," or "transportation," for getting the energy message from master to student. (The concept is similar to using acupuncture needles as a communications vehicle to move Qi from the TCM practitioner to the patient. The needle is the conveyance. The success of the treatment depends on *who* uses the needle.) The student then uses this message to help restore and reenergize the function of his or her internal Qi.

The first type of Qigong is like having your computer professor teach you how to write a program that can help improve your health. Using his instructions, you must write your own program and then use it by yourself in your personal computer. There are no other connections. How well you can apply this program now depends on you and your own intuition. With the second type of Qigong, the professor first reveals to you the principles and theories of the entire health program; then he teaches you how to apply this knowledge and how to write your own special program. Then instead of making you do the work of writing the computer program yourself, he surprises you and gives you a gift. He transfers a copy of a first-rate, time-tested program to you, and then allows you to link your own personal computer to the mainframe where all the knowledge of this health program resides. In this latter system, the energy connection between master and student is far more important than postures. Using this kind of program saves enormous energy, which can then be directed toward self-healing.

This type of Qigong is very special because the master can use any object to pass healing energy and messages to his or her patient. For instance, they can give a gift that carries this kind of message. The patient can then wear the gift, like a ring or necklace, and receive more healing benefits. The master can also use art, like painting, drawing or calligraphy. In this case, the master will give the patient a special piece of art to take home. Sometimes, a highly skilled master can use music for healing. This music is not like New Age meditation music, because when the master creates it, healing energy is basically "channeled" through him or her for a very specific healing purpose, or even for a specific person and their condition.

Sadly, it is very difficult to find this kind of Qigong master today. From my experience, it's also difficult to find patients with an open mind who can accept this type of energy treatment. If, however, the patient can open her mind, this is really the highest level of healing she can receive. This way she is being treated directly through healing Qi that reaches deeply into her body and mind. If she's treated with herbs, or acupuncture or acupressure, a transfer vehicle is involved. When that happens, just like a battery, there is an automatic step down or reduction in the percentage of the Qi transmitted. Also, this type of treatment requires that the practitioner and patient form a deep energy bond.

Why are these kinds of Qigong masters hard to find? First, these masters must have been taught by a skilled master. Their master must have trained them to discover this special gift. Second, even if they are lucky enough to meet a high-level Qigong master, if they haven't been born to receive this gift, then the gift will never go beyond these masters. Think about how most parents would like to pass along their special talents to their children. But even if a parent is a brilliant musician, he or she cannot make his or her child into one. The child has to have both the innate talent and the ability to receive the parent's gift. This gift is beyond technique and beyond words. In its simplest terms, it is an energy transfer.

The *Wu Ming* Meridian Therapy for weight management in this book falls into the second category of Qigong. I have selected the set of ten Qigong movements that follow for their ability to help stimulate your Qi to flow freely in the meridians that affect your liver, spleen, kidney, and lung—organs directly related to weight problems. They can also help you reawaken your natural healing ability. Remember, the more you practice, the more you will gain. One of our participants shared this story with us.

Like a lot of Americans, I've been through a number of different weight loss and health programs. I thought I understood the body's self-healing nature pretty well before I began this program. Now, I have to say, I experience it much differently. Through daily practice of various parts of the program, a switch went on one day and it all made sense in a new and wonderful way. Practicing Wu Ming *Meridian Therapy is one of the most important parts of my day. I stopped working out during the program to see if what Dr. Lu said about it was true for me and it is. I was much stronger and much firmer than when I went to the gym! Although I've always had trouble losing weight, I lost twelve pounds and nine inches overall during the program and wasn't hungry at all. My digestive problems, including mild colitis, improved immeasurably. I under-*

*stand now how my past food choices aggravated my prob-
lems even though they followed conventional diet advice.
The mental clarity I have is remarkable. I try to start each
day smiling from my heart (a longevity practice that I
learned in the program). What a difference The Dragon's
Way has made in my life.*

VALERIE R., 50-YEAR-OLD PHYSICAL EDUCATION TEACHER

THE DRAGON'S WAY *WU MING* MERIDIAN THERAPY

Before you begin, here are some simple guidelines for practicing
The Dragon's Way energy movements:

1. Practice in comfortable clothing.
2. Practice the entire program of ten movements at least
   once a day. The set should take about twenty minutes.
3. Try to practice at the same time each day. A good time
   to increase Qi is from 11:00 A.M. to 1:00 P.M. and from
   5:00 P.M. to 7:00 P.M.
4. It is very beneficial also to practice during the full moon,
   as well as seasonal transitions like the winter solstice,
   spring equinox, etc. Your birthday and time of birth and
   your parents' birthdays are also good times.
5. Practice the movements separately whenever you can.
   When you do this, you'll gain the most benefit from practicing them individually for at least five minutes.
6. *Wu Ming* Meridian Therapy requires no special breathing techniques, so breathe naturally. Do not hold your
   breath or try to create a special breathing pattern.
7. There is no special mental focus. Try to remain peaceful
   and concentrate on what you are doing. Before you
   begin, you can try some slow, deep breathing. Then give

yourself an overall positive message of self-healing. Do not focus on a particular organ or meridian.

8. When you reach a certain level in this ancient self-healing system, you will notice that the Qigong energy itself will cut off your thoughts and help you enter a timeless space where you can help heal yourself.

9. Do not practice when you are very hungry, after a big meal, after sex, or if you are very tired.

1. The Dragon's Toe Dance

Stand with your feet shoulder-width apart. Start with your left side. Raise your left heel up and bend your knee. Your weight should be on the ball of your foot. Now, slowly rotate your leg outward. Make sure you feel your ankle, knee and hip joints turning together.

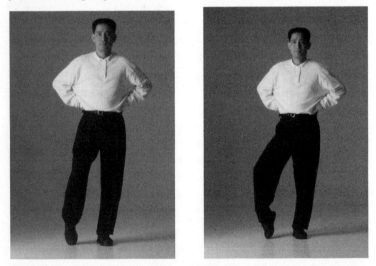

Now count slowly: 1-2-3-4; 2-2-3-4; 3-2-3-4; 4-2-3-4. Do this set three times. Twelve times equals about one minute per side.

Now, change to your right side and do the same thing.

2. The Dragon Kicks Forward

Stand comfortably with your feet should-width apart. Start with your left side. Kick out gently with your heel and let your whole leg stretch out. Do not kick too high or too fast. Remember, these are meridian stretches and you want to feel this stretch through the back of your leg. Each kick out is one count. Do three sets of four, counting in the same manner as in the first movement: 1-2-3-4; 2-2-3-4; 3-2-3-4; 4-2-3-4. Now stop and change to your right side. Use the same count. (If you find that your balance is unsteady, hold onto a chair, or table, etc. As your Qi increases you will find it easier to perform this movement without holding onto anything.)

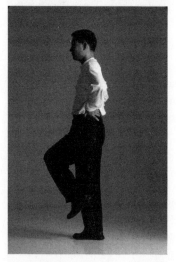
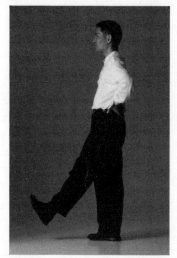

3. The Dragon's Twist

Stand comfortably with your arms at your sides. Start with your left side. Make sure your weight is on your left side and your right hip bone turns forward. This is a kind of gentle swinging motion where your whole body twists from one side to the other. Do six sets of four, counting in the same manner as in the first movement: 1-2-3-4; 2-2-3-4; 3-2-3-4; 4-2-3-4.

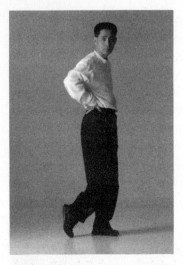
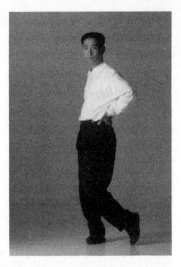

4. The Dragon's Punch

Again, stand with your feet shoulder-width apart. Start off with your left leg. Step forward gently and easily with your heel coming down first. At the same time you step forward with your left foot, gently punch your right hand forward straight out in front of you in a corkscrew motion so that your fist "eye" ends up turning downward. Alternate this with your right foot and left arm, punching in the same way. Do ten sets of four in total, counting as above. Each punch out and back should take four counts: 1-2-3-4; 2-2-3-4; 3-2-3-4; 4-2-3-4, and so on.

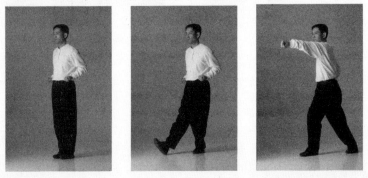

5. The Dragon Looks at His Tail

Stand with your feet shoulder-width apart. Start with your left leg. Step forward with this leg and as you do extend your right arm backwards with your palm turned up. Turn your head and slowly look back at your right palm. Now alternate this movement with the right leg and the left arm. Remember to look back down your arm and see your palm turned upward. Do ten sets of four, counting as above.

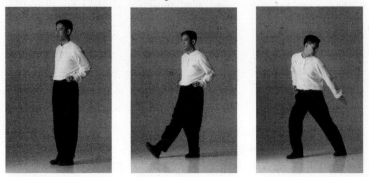

6. The Dragon Taps His Foot

Stand with your feet shoulder-width apart. Put your weight on the left side. Stretch your right leg out to the side, lift it up a few inches and bring it back down in the same place, hitting the inside of your right foot against the floor. Alternate with the right side. Do three sets of four on each side, counting as above.

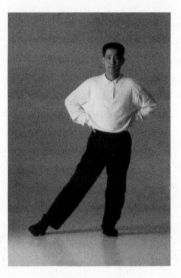

7. Rocking the Baby Dragon

Stand with your feet shoulder-width apart. As if you were going to rock a baby, put your arms together in front of you, leaving a little space between your hands. Now slowly swing your arms up to the left side first and look up at your elbow at the same time. Swing your arms up to the right side in a rocking motion. Swing from left to right and do four sets of six, counting as above.

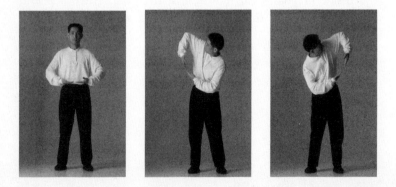

8. The Dragon Kicks Backward

Stand with your feet shoulder-width apart. Put your weight on your right foot and start with your left leg. Kick the left leg straight back, gently leading with your heel. Do not kick too high or too fast. Repeat with your right foot. Do three sets of four, counting as above. (See note in movement #2 above.)

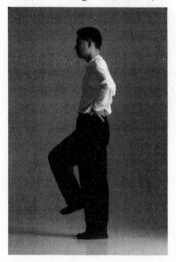 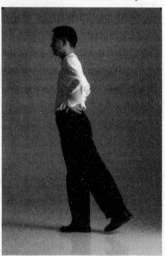

9. The Dragon Rises From the Ocean

Stand with your feet shoulder-width apart. Make a fist and hold each fist tightly at your side with your elbows bent. Breathe in deeply. When you breathe in, you are bringing Qi into your body. Exhale deeply. When you breathe out, imagine that you are pushing fat and water out of your body. In a gentle rhythm that goes "Breathe in . . . breathe out . . . ," breathe in and out twenty times, counting one inhalation and exhalation as one breath. Do not rush your breathing.

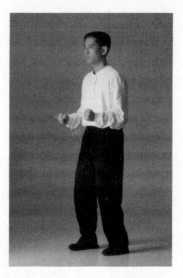

10. The Dragon Stands Between Heaven and Earth

Stand with your feet shoulder-width apart. Relax and remain comfortable. Make sure your knees are bent slightly. With your hands hanging loosely in front of you, make a fist with your thumbs pointing toward each other. With your fist and thumbs in this position, bend your elbows and raise your arms to chest level. Your fists and thumbs will be pointing toward each other. Close your eyes and imagine you are the Dragon standing between heaven and earth. Feel this power. Practice by standing in this position for at least three minutes; longer is better. In fact, the longer you can hold this posture, the more healing benefits you will gain. Open your eyes slowly and try to keep this good feeling with you at all times.

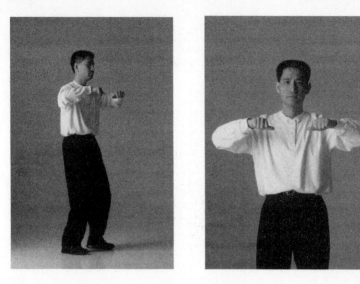

Remember that these ancient secrets of energy healing can help you change your life. The Dragon's Way is now your way.

WU MING MERIDIAN THERAPY: YOUR DAILY PRACTICE CHART

1. The Dragon's Toe Dance
2. The Dragon Kicks Forward
3. The Dragon's Twist
4. The Dragon's Punch
5. The Dragon Looks at His Tail
6. The Dragon Taps His Foot
7. Rocking the Baby Dragon
8. The Dragon Kicks Backward
9. The Dragon Rises From the Ocean
10. The Dragon Stands Between Heaven and Earth

You can record each movement you do for each day of the program on the following chart. Record any additional practice time under "extra."

WU MING MERIDIAN THERAPY PRACTICE RECORD

DAY	1	2	3	4	5	6	7	8	9	10	EXTRA
1											
2											
3											
4											
5											
6											
7											
8											
9											
10											
11											
12											
13											
14											
15											
16											
17											
18											
19											
20											

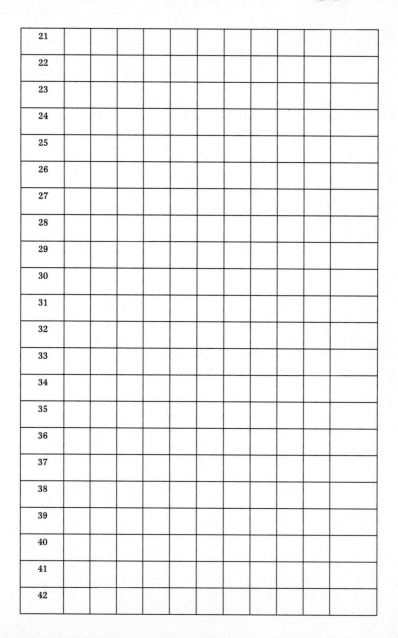

21											
22											
23											
24											
25											
26											
27											
28											
29											
30											
31											
32											
33											
34											
35											
36											
37											
38											
39											
40											
41											
42											

PART II

TAKING OFF TWELVE POUNDS AND EIGHT INCHES IN SIX WEEKS THE DRAGON'S WAY

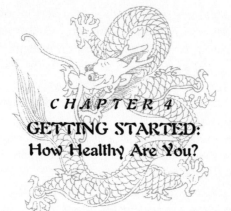

CHAPTER 4
GETTING STARTED:
How Healthy Are You?

OUR bodies are born with an innate intelligence that governs their ability to self-heal. Our self-healing process is fueled by Qi. If your Qi is strong and balanced and you take good care of yourself, your own energy system will, by and large, be able to regulate itself. By middle age, however, our bodies are showing the effects of years of stress, possibly unhealthy lifestyle habits, and our Qi has declined and gotten out of balance.

I find that many women are drawn to The Dragon's Way and are very satisfied with the way it makes them feel. Most are in the thirty-nine to fifty-plus age range, although we've had a number of participants who were older (eighty years old) and younger (nineteen to thirty years old). The men tend to be in their mid-thirties and older. If you're one of the millions of women who are experiencing perimenopause, The Dragon's Way can be particularly helpful. Your body's Qi and the function of your organs are just starting to decline. At this early stage, it may be easy to tune up your system. Acupuncture or herbs, alone or in combination, might well bring quick relief from symptoms. If they do, be sure not to stop treatment too soon. Even if symptoms seem to disappear, the function of your

 63

organs will still need support. It's a good idea to continue treatment for a while so you can be sure you've addressed the source of the problem. If you're taking herbs, for example, keep taking them even if you seem to be fine. These herbs are designed to help your organs function better so that you can heal yourself. Then you can gradually switch from herbal therapy to self-healing with foods.

If you're dealing with weight problems, you can now understand where they come from and why. You may also want to combine The Dragon's Way with other TCM healing methods, including classical Chinese herbs and acupuncture.

If you've been overweight for a long time or if you have a lot of weight to lose, you must be patient with yourself. One thing to remember is that once you've healed the root problem, you will be free to eat whatever you want in a balanced way because your body's self-regulating and self-healing ability will have been restored.

When you recover your own healing ability, I hope you will recognize that your old over-stressed lifestyle patterns were the cause of your weight problem. I hope The Dragon's Way will teach you how to take good care of yourself the TCM way. If you feel better, you may do what some of my Western patients do. So happy to feel well again, they think they can resume their old life. If you do, watch out. I tell them, "I don't understand this. Why are you trying to go back to the lifestyle that caused your symptoms in the first place? You've learned to do things differently now. Trust this program."

Usually, I make a joke with my participants and tell them, "The secret of living a long healthy life is—do nothing!" They laugh and say, "I want to do something." Again I tell them, "Do nothing. That is the best 'something' you can do." They say, "You have a lot of courage telling people in this culture that they ought to do nothing, especially in New York City." The greatest way to heal and to live a long healthy life is to understand the value of not being in motion twenty-four hours a day and of having a calm and peaceful heart.

SELF-HEALING TCM CHECKLISTS

The following checklists are based on the TCM principles and theories discussed throughout this book. The questions and answers can help you heal yourself and get to a balanced state of health. TCM states that when Qi runs smoothly through the meridians and the organs work in harmony, there is no way for disease or illness to enter your body, not even cancer! I want to point out again that the *Nei Jing,* the most famous TCM medical text, stated this principle more than two thousand years ago. This principle has been practiced for much longer than that. To this day, it has never been contradicted or overturned as a way of understanding the optimum state of health. Please use these checklists to guide you to new habits and a more healthy lifestyle.

An essential part of a TCM prevention program, these checklists can help alert you to unhealthy lifestyle habits that you should eliminate and minor health problems that you can address to prevent them from becoming catastrophic illnesses, like breast or other kinds of cancer.

Work with these self-healing checklists to create your initial health profile. As you perform *Wu Ming* Meridian Therapy, follow The Dragon's Way Eating for Healing plan, and make daily lifestyle changes, you will gradually notice a difference in your well-being. You will know that the program is working. Congratulations! You are beginning to awaken the power to heal yourself!

If you answer yes to more than three of the questions in any one checklist, you should know that your lifestyle habits can eventually cause you physical problems, such as excess weight. These problems will emerge first as a Qi dysfunction. It is critical to understand that if these problems are left uncorrected, they can progress to much deeper physical problems. Don't let this happen to you. Take these signs seriously.

I have set up six separate checklists. Look over the answers and, where possible, try to make the necessary changes suggested. You can coordinate this knowledge with everything you've learned in The Dragon's Way. With this ancient wisdom, and these unique TCM techniques and tools, you can take control of and responsibility for your healing process. You now have the gift of a lifetime—for a lifetime!

I. SELF-HEALING CHECKLIST FOR EATING HABITS

Taking Care of Your Digestive System

1. Do you eat barbecued or fried foods often?

2. Do you always drink ice-cold drinks or ice water?

3. Do you eat raw vegetables or eat at salad bars frequently?

4. Do you get a headache after you have a meal?

5. Do you experience stomach distension whenever you eat?

6. Do you have a stomachache after you eat, particularly after eating cold or dairy foods?

7. Do you always burp or pass gas after you eat?

8. Do you always have loose stool after you eat?

9. Do you drink too much alcohol? More than two glasses a day?

10. Do you have food allergies?

ANSWER SECTION ON EATING HABITS

A function disorder of your stomach will cause Qi to stagnate in your stomach meridians. From an energy standpoint, it is essential to keep your stomach functioning well. If you are a woman, this is particularly important information. You should know that 50 percent of breast cancer cases develop in the upper outer quadrant of the left breast, a location TCM understands as being related to stomach meridians. Therefore, keeping this organ functioning properly is essential to keeping Qi flowing freely in this critical breast area.

1. Barbecued or fried foods can cause a stomach function disorder by creating an excess of heat in this organ. This condition of internal heat can be compared with the kind of heat emitted by a compost heap. It is a kind of intense, inner smoldering, which then prevents the stomach from performing its normal job—one aspect of which is to work in harmony with the liver. According to TCM, the stomach and the liver must have a healthy partnership to digest food well. If these two organs cannot work in harmony, you will not get enough nutrition or Qi from the foods you eat.

2. The stomach's very nature is warmth-loving. Warmth then is the natural law upon which it operates. Your stomach "loves" to receive warm things like soup, warm drinks like tea, cocoa, etc. If you constantly eat or drink cold foods or beverages, you can unbalance the stomach's natural function and cause it to perform sluggishly. Women who frequently eat and drink cold things during the menstrual cycle should know that this can draw cold energy into the liver and uterus, which, in turn, can cause cramps, an irregular cycle, or other types of female problems. Everyone on The Dragon's Way should try to stick with warm foods and foods with a warm essence like ginger, cinnamon, fennel, etc.

3. Many people in Western cultures believe that eating raw vegetables provides better nutrition. TCM believes that raw vegetables have a cold essence that can impair the stomach's natural function. Even though you may get a little more nutrition from raw food, you will use up more Qi to digest it. If you cook a vegetable slightly, you may lose a little bit of nutrition, but you will save a lot of Qi that could better be diverted to healing and protecting your stomach function.

4. The stomach meridians run up through the forehead area. Generally speaking, headaches in the front of the forehead that occur after a meal indicate a stomach Qi deficiency because the stomach is drawing on too much Qi to digest its food.

5. Stomach distension means that you are suffering from a stomach Qi deficiency. It also indicates that your liver is not working in harmony with your stomach. As we've noted, digesting food well depends on a good partnership between these two organs. Stomach distension means they are not supporting each other's function. Too much stress usually causes this kind of discomfort.

6. As indicated in number (2), the stomach's nature is warmth-loving. If you get a stomachache after you eat cold foods, your stomach Qi has become unbalanced and is now too cold. This is a signal that you should change your eating habits immediately and switch to giving the stomach warm foods or foods with warm essence (such as ginger, cinnamon, scallion, clove, and fennel). They can help relieve this kind of stomachache.

7. Again, burping or passing gas after you eat indicates that the stomach's Qi is deficient. Your organ does not have enough Qi to manage its assigned task of digestion. If this happens after you eat raw vegetables, cheese or other dairy products, or when you're under stress, it is a sign that your stomach and liver's partnership is shaky. Again, this is a symptom that they cannot function in harmony with each other.

8. Loose stool after eating means that the stomach and spleen both have a Qi deficiency. Since the stomach and spleen are partner organs operating as one organ system, this is an important condition to fix. Your whole digestive system is weak. Avoid cold foods; substitute warm foods.

9. Excess alcohol will cause the liver's Qi to stagnate. If the liver's Qi stagnates long enough, it will affect the stomach's Qi and cause a disruption in communication between the two organs. Again, here is a lifestyle habit that has the potential to seriously

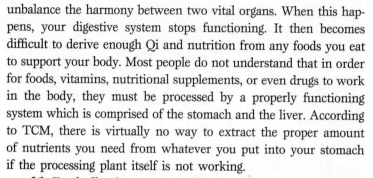

unbalance the harmony between two vital organs. When this happens, your digestive system stops functioning. It then becomes difficult to derive enough Qi and nutrition from any foods you eat to support your body. Most people do not understand that in order for foods, vitamins, nutritional supplements, or even drugs to work in the body, they must be processed by a properly functioning system which is comprised of the stomach and the liver. According to TCM, there is virtually no way to extract the proper amount of nutrients you need from whatever you put into your stomach if the processing plant itself is not working.

10. Food allergies are an indication that your stomach Qi is low or deficient. It also means that your stomach cannot work in harmony with the liver, spleen, and gallbladder. Many people, in an attempt to address their allergies, gradually cut out one food after another in their diet in the hope of relief. Sometimes, I see patients who are basically down to eating rice cakes and water because they have become so sensitive. They are so focused on believing that their problem is caused externally by the foods themselves, that they are literally shocked when I tell them it is their stomach that is the problem. Changing your diet alone does not get to the root cause of food allergies. Avoiding cold foods, raw foods, and ice-cold liquids can help significantly. Adding warm foods and foods with a warm essence like ginger and cinnamon can also help. Start changing your diet today using the information in this book. If you suffer from food allergies, this step can make a big difference in the state of your health. Practicing *Wu Ming* Meridian Therapy can help by increasing Qi and relieving Qi stagnation.

II. SELF-HEALING CHECKLIST ON SLEEP HABITS

1. Do you have difficulty going to sleep each night?
2. Do you wake up at the same time each night? What time?

3. Do the same dreams recur frequently?
4. Do you have nightmares?
5. Do you experience night sweats?
6. Do you go to bed after midnight?
7. Do you eat a big meal just before you go to sleep?
8. Do you have to take a sleeping pill or other drug to sleep soundly?
9. Do you get up to urinate frequently during the night?

ANSWER SECTION ON SLEEP HABITS

Sleep is the natural state in which your physical body and its energy system both take a rest and regenerate themselves. During this time, your body's Qi can recharge itself—much like a battery. If you sleep well, your body is ready to go with a new charge. If you sleep poorly and wake often, you have less Qi to get through your day. TCM examines your dreaming to diagnose the quality of your sleep. For example, if your body is in deep harmony, your sleep will be quite deep, and you should not consciously remember your dreams. You still dream, but these dreams are not accessible to your conscious mind. (TCM also uses dream interpretation to understand the condition of Qi in your various organs.)

1. If you often have difficulty falling asleep, generally speaking, your spleen and heart Qi or energies are deficient. This means these two organ systems are not functioning in harmony. Balance is an important step toward harmony. The state of harmony is the result of one dynamic system wherein there is a smooth, automatic, unconscious exchange of energy. In this instance, your spleen and heart are out of sync. Your heart is not peaceful enough to contain your spirit and you cannot calm down long enough to fall asleep. If you toss and turn during sleep, the cause is the same.

2. TCM theory states that Universal Qi changes every two hours. The Qi in your organs also changes every two hours.

Like a giant gear, if your body's Qi cannot match or mesh with Universal Qi changes, then many different kinds of physical discomforts will develop. TCM recognizes these conditions as biorhythm disorders. For example, Qi changes start with the lung, which is "on duty" or in charge of the body, from 3:00 to 5:00 A.M. If your lung's Qi has a problem, then you might find yourself waking up during this two-hour window. Or, you might wake up with a physical problem like a cough during these hours. Here are the two-hour periods in which each organ's Qi is in charge:

Lung	3:00 A.M.–5:00 A.M.
Large intestine	5:00 A.M.–7:00 A.M.
Spleen	7:00 A.M.–9:00 A.M.
Stomach	9:00 A.M.–11:00 A.M.
Heart	11:00 A.M.–1:00 P.M.
Small intestine	1:00 P.M.–3:00 P.M.
Bladder	3:00 P.M.–5:00 P.M.
Kidney	5:00 P.M.–7:00 P.M.
Pericardium	7:00 P.M.–9:00 P.M.
Triple warmer*	9:00 P.M.–11:00 P.M.
Gallbladder	11:00 P.M.–1:00 A.M.
Liver	1:00 A.M.–3:00 A.M.

*In TCM, the triple warmer is a meridian without a specific organ. It covers the upper body above the heart, the middle body from below the heart to the navel, and the lower body from the navel to the feet.

3. Dream diagnosis or interpretation is one tool TCM uses to understand a patient's physical condition. Problems that are Qi- or energy-related in the internal organs show up in different kinds of dreams. For instance, if your heart Qi is deficient, you might feel yourself falling out of the sky, or off a tall building. If you have a kidney Qi deficiency, you might have dreams that are connected to drowning or being under water, or being in a boat that is capsizing. Or, you might find yourself being fearful and hiding from something in your dreams. If you refer to The Five Element Theory Chart on page (133), you can see where this insight comes from. Water is the element of the kidney and fear is its ruling emotion. You can gain more insight into your dreams by studying this ancient blueprint. If you always see yourself arguing or fighting or things are destroyed in your dreams, then you might have a parasite, or these could be signals that your internal problem might be worsening. These are all classical Chinese dream interpretations.

4. Generally speaking, nightmares indicate a liver Qi deficiency; nightmares that contain images of people chasing you, wanting to kill you, or harm you usually indicate a problem with unbalanced liver Qi. If you have these kinds of nightmares, your physical liver organ may be fine, but the way it is functioning is definitely in need of attention. If these dreams occur frequently, your body is sending you strong signals that the liver needs your help. According to TCM, the liver is the most important organ for women's health. For men, it is the kidney. If you're a woman, I recommend paying serious attention to these kinds of internal warnings. If Qi stagnates in the liver or this organ becomes completely out of balance, you are looking head on at the root cause of breast cancer.

5. The body has two types of Qi—yin Qi and yang Qi. Sweating at night indicates that your body's yin Qi is deficient. This means that at nighttime, your body's Qi cannot control the normal opening and closing of your skin pores. One of the key principles of TCM is that both types of Qi—yin and yang—must work in harmony. Daytime Qi is considered yang; nighttime Qi, yin. If you have more physical discomfort in the daytime, your body's yang Qi is deficient or is not sufficient enough to handle normal daytime tasks. The reverse is true if your problems occur at night.

6. It is important to understand this from a Qi perspective. Your body enters its yin Qi phase after midnight; at this time your body's yang Qi makes its way deep into your internal

organs with the goal of rejuvenating them. To remain in harmony, your body should follow nature's way. If you stay up past midnight, you are working against nature's cycle. Your body will spend more than twice the amount of Qi for every hour you're awake just to stay awake. To save your Qi or vital energy and prevent disease or illness, it's important to follow nature's cycle. This is also important when you're trying to lose weight. For women, this is an especially key lifestyle habit to change before you reach perimenopause or menopause.

7. Many people in the United States eat a big dinner and then go to sleep. This often causes sleep problems. TCM understands that insomnia is related to different types of stomach Qi dysfunctions. When you eat a big meal, the stomach's Qi will overfunction or work too hard. By overworking, it can fall out of harmony with the liver and heart. (Refer to The Five Element Chart to see the kinds of relationships these organs share). That's why some people feel heartburn after a big meal; however, the root cause is often a stomach Qi dysfunction. Healthy eating means that you should only eat to about 70 to 75 percent capacity of your stomach. Eating too much before bedtime can cause your stomach to use extra Qi to function all night long just to digest what you've eaten, when it should be conserving this Qi for self-healing and resting. Here again is another simple, yet effective, way in which you can build up your Qi and not waste it.

8. TCM understands that sleeping well means your body is functioning in harmony. If you frequently or always rely on sleeping pills or drugs, your body cannot function in harmony. Also, these substances might be hiding a deeper internal problem that needs to be fixed. I recommend finding other natural ways to help you sleep better. Drinking a glass of celery juice before bedtime might help. Also, practice Qigong or try to meditate for twenty minutes or so before going to bed.

9. Urinary frequency during the night indicates a kidney Qi deficiency. This means that your kidney cannot send its part-

ner organ, your bladder, the right messages and enough Qi to hold your urine throughout the night. This problem can appear during menopause and cause fatigue. *The Dragon Kicks Backward* (#8) in the *Wu Ming* Meridian Therapy series can help you strengthen your kidney Qi. If this condition occurs during or after cancer treatments, it means your body's overall Qi has dropped significantly. If so, I recommend frequent practice.

III. SELF-HEALING CHECKLIST ON WORK HABITS

1. Do you work in or around high power electrical areas, or where there is radiation, such as a microwave?

2. Do you work with chemicals?

3. Do you like your job?

4. Do you work under chronic stress?

5. Do you work straight through your day without taking a lunch break?

6. Do you work and eat at the same time?

7. Do you get along with the people you work with?

8. Is your work area comfortable and healthy?

ANSWER SECTION ON WORK HABITS

Your daily lifestyle has a tremendous impact on the state of your health. Understanding how to shape your work experience so that it supports your health and your ability to lose weight is a very important aspect of self-healing. Many people spend more than eight hours a day at their workplace. While you may not be able to change your workplace itself, you can begin to pay attention to any negative effects it has on you and begin to change your responses to them.

I remind Dragon's Way participants that it is their old lifestyle that has contributed to their current weight problems. I advise them to let go of the stresses that filled their old life and create a new calmer, more peaceful one. I also urge you too to change your habits and your emotional responses to the many stresses in your daily life if you truly want to heal the root cause of your overweight symptoms.

1. Electrical fields can interfere with or change your body's own electrical field. New scientific work with bioelectromagnetics at Stanford University in California shows that even very subtle frequencies, far below what was previously considered safe, can create cellular changes. Electrical fields can cause a dysfunction in the flow of Qi through your meridians. They also have the ability to cause a serious Qi deficiency. The stronger the field, the worse the effect. If you work around areas with a lot of radiation, your energy field can also be easily disrupted and unbalanced by this kind of energy force. If you are continually exposed to these kinds of energies, you are at risk for compromising your own self-healing ability.

2. Certain kinds of chemicals can either directly or indirectly cause cancer. Even if you don't touch the chemical itself, simply smelling it can disrupt the smooth and healthy functioning of your lung. How is this possible? Remember that, according to TCM theory, the sense organ associated with the lung is the nose. Additionally, the lung controls the health of the skin. If your lung function is interrupted or unbalanced, then your skin can be affected.

3. Because you spend the largest part of your day at your job, you invest a lot of emotional, physical, mental, and spiritual Qi there. If you don't like your job, but you must keep it, then your mind and spirit are in conflict and under constant pressure. This condition can cause internal Qi stagnation in any organ or meridian. This is the earliest stage of an energy imbalance within the body.

4. Stress takes a deadly toll on the liver. If your liver function is out of balance, then you might experience physical discomfort in the form of symptoms such as stomach distension or bloating, nail problems, and itchy and/or red eyes, and for women, PMS and menstrual disorders. If the liver continues to be stressed over time, this condition can lead to function disorders of your other major organs, the stomach, kidney, heart, and lung. It is vital to find a healthy way to deal with the stress in your life. It is important not to absorb the negative energy of stress into your own energy system, but find productive ways to let it go. If you live with chronic stress, especially in your job, think very carefully about how you can change this health-robbing situation, and, if you cannot, whether you are really willing to give away your health in return for a paycheck.

TCM has a time-honored and very successful way to alleviate anger: smash eggs! In fact, buy a dozen eggs (a pretty inexpensive way to let out stress) and smash them all. If you live in an apartment, you can throw the eggs against the shower wall or the bathtub. Believe it or not, this simple act can help you physically and emotionally relieve a lot of anger and stress. Many of my patients laugh and say to me, "Why didn't you tell me to buy two dozen eggs! I loved smashing these eggs and I really felt a major shift within me by doing this. What an amazing experience." No eggs? Try smashing raw potatoes with your feet (shoes on!). Or, in a safe place, break glass bottles. Releasing negative energy can definitely help you heal the root cause of a number of stress-related and other problems; the results are remarkable.

Acupuncture, Taiji, Yoga, and meditation, as well as certain classical Chinese herbal formulas, can help relieve stress. Our *Wu Ming* Meridian Therapy movements are especially effective at helping you reduce chronic stress in your life. Beyond this, they can also help you deepen your spiritual connection with the Universe and its vibration of unconditional love.

5. Because of the busy lives people lead today, they often work long, stress-filled hours, sometimes forgetting to stop for lunch. This causes the body to expend or burn up extra Qi for daily activity. When this happens, your body is forced to draw on its irreplaceable kidney Qi to keep going. This is not a good situation because it should be running instead on the Qi of your rechargeable stomach energy to get through the day.

Not eating healthy foods at regular intervals will cause a stomach function disorder that could eventually lead to digestive system problems later like food allergies, bloating after eating, and weight gain. Again, continuing this unhealthy habit can lead to more serious digestive problems when the stomach becomes unable to extract nutrition from the things you eat. Function problems of the stomach itself or problems of Qi stagnation in the stomach's meridian could disrupt the healthy flow of Qi through the stomach meridians.

6. Working and eating at the same time is not a healthy habit. If you make a regular practice of doing this, then your digestive system will not get sufficient Qi to do its job. You may not be able to gain maximum nutrition from the food you're eating while you're working. If you continually work and eat at the same time, you can literally upset or unbalance the normal healthy functioning of your stomach. Then, one of the problems you may eventually experience is stomachaches after eating. Here is one daily activity that you can change for the better to help yourself heal. Even if it's only fifteen or twenty minutes, take some time for yourself and eat your meal in peace and quiet. Do not answer the phone, or hold a meeting, or try to balance your checkbook at this time. Just take the time to eat slowly and thoughtfully. Keeping this organ and its meridians functioning well is true prevention.

7. While you don't have to love the people you work with, it's very important to have a harmonious work experience. Otherwise, your body will spend extra Qi to deal with emotional issues on a daily basis. This emotional discomfort can cause a function disorder of one or more of your five major organs. Look at The Five Element Theory Chart and study which emotions can affect which organs. According to TCM theories, holding unbalanced and/or negative emotions in the body for a long time can lead to Qi stagnation and eventually cause serious physical damage.

I want to emphasize that it is not experiencing an emotion that is damaging (unless, of course, it is sudden and severe). We're all human and we experience a range of emotions each and every day. It is chronically holding negative emotions that causes health problems. To remain well, it is important to find productive ways to release excess emotions from your body and become good at "letting things go." Try to follow nature's lead and "go with the flow."

8. Again, since you spend so many of your waking hours in the workplace, it is very important to create harmony in your environment to the best of your ability. This way your body does not have to divert extra Qi just to maintain its normal functions. Even a few small changes can help you conserve your Qi. When a plant flowers, it is at the peak of its own Qi. Try to bring a fresh flower often into your workspace to experience this special energy. This kind of "live" message can help your body recall its own healing ability. Place a healthy plant near your computer. When your eyes become tired, change your field of vision to the plant. This can help you relieve eyestrain and help keep your vision healthy.

Everyone can take a few short breaks throughout the workday. When you do, close your eyes and breathe slowly and deeply. Let everything go; do not focus on any problems or physical sensations or emotions. I tell my patients that even a few minutes done occasionally throughout the day can really help them recharge their energy base. From my experience, many short meditations can produce the same effect as a full twenty minutes of meditation. Getting into this habit can change your life and help you accumulate Qi over the course of the day that you'll need to help heal the condition of excess weight. Don't miss these simple opportunities to really help yourself.

IV. SELF-HEALING CHECKLIST ON EMOTIONAL STABILITY

1. Do you have depression? Do you take medication for depression?
2. Do you suffer from anger continually?
3. Do you cry easily and often?
4. Do you suffer from anxiety or panic attacks?
5. Is it hard for you to make decisions?
6. Do you worry all the time?
7. Are you under a lot of stress for continued periods of time?
8. Do you suffer from frequent mood swings?
9. Do negative events from the past continue to bother you today?

ANSWER SECTION ON EMOTIONAL STABILITY

TCM does not believe emotions are something that occurs only in your mind or in your thoughts. It identifies five specific emotions that, if experienced excessively, have the ability to destroy the healthy functioning of an organ. As we've seen in The Five Element Theory, TCM believes the liver is related to anger—too much anger held for a long period of time can unbalance healthy liver function. Overthinking or constant worry will cause stomach and spleen function problems, sometimes manifesting as a loss of appetite or excess water retention, respectively. Healthy lung function can be destroyed by chronic sadness or grief. A continual state of fear will compromise the kidney's regular function. And too much happiness will ultimately cause a heart function problem. If you want to remain healthy, you must keep your emotions in a state of balance.

1. TCM understands depression as a disharmony between liver and spleen Qi. If you use drugs to help alleviate depression, you may have a temporary lifting of the condition, but the underlying root cause is still there. Like pushing a ball under water, sooner or later the problem will pop up again unless this root cause is fixed. TCM understands that treatment of this problem means addressing both the internal Qi imbalances and the emotional reactions to external factors that cause this illness. It is important to identify why and how this problem has come about. Although drugs for depression have helped many people through many difficult times, it is important to recognize that they can eventually cause liver and stomach function problems.

2. Anger will cause a liver function disorder. Because the liver is responsible for the smooth flow of Qi and blood throughout the body, a liver function disorder can also cause other organs to become out of balance. I see a lot of patients who believe they are not angry people and have dealt with their anger over certain situations. If you ask them if they are angry, they will tell you no. However, when we begin to talk about something that bothers them, they exhibit all the signs of anger, even though, in some cases, the event was long ago.

3. Crying is related to the lung function and sometimes the stomach and spleen functions. Crying all the time can weaken the Qi of all three organs. They will then not be strong enough to keep their ruling emotions stable (be sure and identify these emotions from The Five Element Theory Chart), nor will they be able to help keep your overall emotional Qi stable.

4. Anxiety and panic attacks are related to deficient kidney Qi. These conditions can also mean that your kidney and heart are not functioning in harmony. Because the kidney is the Qi foundation for the entire body, the best way to address these conditions is to treat the root cause by strengthening kidney Qi with classical Chinese herbs.

5. TCM understands that the gallbladder rules the body's decision-making capability. If your gallbladder Qi is deficient, or the gallbladder itself has a function disorder, you might have a hard time making decisions. If your gallbladder has been removed, you might also find—especially as you get older—that making decisions becomes difficult. Even though your physical gallbladder may be removed, remember that its meridian still runs in your body. I remind my patients who have had any organ or organs removed that they are different now. They must take very good care of themselves to remain healthy. I urge you to do the same.

Sometimes, gallbladder problems are also related to a liver function disorder. Remember that these two organs share an energy relationship. That is, they are partner organs that are connected and communicate with each other via Qi. If you're always under a lot of stress, or if your liver does not function smoothly with this companion organ, or with the other organs, then gallbladder function will be impaired. Also, if you have digestive problems, such as difficulty eating protein or dairy products, the root problem can lie with the relationship between the gallbladder and the liver.

6. Constant worry can cause spleen and stomach function disorders. If that happens, your digestive system will be affected. Your body will not be able to extract enough nutrition from what you eat, you might experience lack of appetite, you might retain water, and your sleep may become disturbed. Conversely, if your spleen Qi becomes weak or deficient, you may worry constantly.

7. Stress is the number one external emotional cause of liver function disorder; anger is the number one internal emotional cause. Unfortunately, many people today are affected by both of these conditions. If a liver function disorder develops, then you're very likely to have a digestive problem. The consequence of this is an internal Qi crisis. When this crisis occurs, your whole body's energy system can become deficient or weak. The body lacks enough power to support everyday life. It starts "running on empty." This, in turn, causes more stress as you become increasingly unable to manage basic daily activities.

Chronic stress can actually be deadly. It can cause serious Qi stagnation in the meridians and causes most of the health problems many women experience. TCM believes that, for women in transition, as long as kidney Qi can be kept strong and liver function can be kept smooth, then menopausal symptoms can be avoided. When stress begins to affect a man deeply, he can experience neck pain, lower back pain, erectile dysfunction, or high blood pressure, among other conditions.

8. If you suffer from frequent mood swings, two key organs are affected. Your liver Qi is stagnating (the concept of stagnation is like that of a compost heap, which generates a kind of smoldering, internal heat that blocks the free flow of Qi) and your kidney Qi is weak or deficient. Acupuncture and Chinese herbs are very successful treatments for these kinds of problems. Taiji, Yoga, meditation, and gaining support from and relating to nature's own Qi by walking slowly and peacefully outdoors can help you regain your emotional balance.

9. As a method of treatment, TCM tries to relieve or unblock Qi stagnation. If you always mull over the past, replay distressful scenes, reflect on past negative events and feelings, hold grudges, or never forgive, sooner or later this stuck Qi, or Qi stagnation, can turn into a physical blockage, like a tumor or cancer. If you want to heal yourself, completely letting things go is the only way to change your body's energy pattern—no matter what problem, the technique is the same. Since liver Qi stagnation is a serious condition, you must learn to truly "let go."

"Letting go" is one of the most important philosophies of TCM, which uses many different techniques to push disease and illness out of the body. These include: treating a cough to expel it from the body instead of suppressing it or using herbs to put a parasite to sleep instead of trying to eject it with harsh chemicals.

V. SELF-HEALING CHECKLIST ON PLEASURE HABITS

1. Do you have to be in constant motion?
2. Do you overeat?

3. Do you smoke?

4. Do you drink too much alcohol? More than two glasses per day?

5. Do you have frequent sex or frequently change sex partners?

6. Do you perform high-impact exercises more than three times a week?

7. Do you take drugs, either prescription or recreational?

8. Do you take birth control pills?

ANSWER SECTION ON PLEASURE HABITS

1. If you're always in constant motion, you are using up a lot of excess Qi to support your physical and emotional needs. The body is much like a car. It needs a rest; at regular intervals it needs its engine turned off and it needs to cool down. Also, like a car battery, the body needs to recharge itself. According to TCM theory, everyone is born with a finite amount of Qi. If you constantly use up large quantities of Qi, it hastens the time when this finite amount is completely depleted; in other words, it's time to die. It may appear that you're accomplishing a lot of things when you're in constant motion, but in reality, you may not be doing the best job, or even the highest quality work. You may be in motion without reason.

If you're one of those people who must be in constant motion, you may also tend to become frustrated more easily. This can unbalance your liver function, which, in turn, can set off a negative cycle that can lead to more serious health problems. When your energy level falls too low or weakens, you are also more vulnerable to getting sick. You do not have an adequate reserve of Qi to heal yourself. Learn to say "enough" and give yourself permission to slow down and make intelligent choices about how to use your time and your Qi.

2. If you continually overeat, you can cause a serious stomach function disorder. Your stomach will become distended; you might experience heartburn. Overeating will also cause your

body to spend much more of its Qi to digest what you've eaten. According to TCM, a stomach dysfunction can also cause insomnia. Often, sleep problems are caused by eating a big meal too late at night. If you have this kind of problem, don't take sleeping pills. Shift your eating habits and avoid eating or drinking too much before bedtime. Healthy eating means eating enough not to feel hungry later. This requires tuning into your body's signals so that you can recognize what a satisfied feeling means for your body. I recommend eating to about 70 percent of the capacity of your stomach. Not eating too much can also improve your mental function by helping you think more clearly and by eliminating a sluggish feeling.

3. Everyone knows that smoking is harmful to your health. Cigarette smoke can not only cause lung cancer by affecting this organ and its meridian, but it will also affect the organs and meridians with which the lung shares an energetic relationship—your large intestine and kidney. Although you may not realize it, smoking can cause large intestine and kidney function disorders. If these organs are out of balance, you will gain weight after you've quit smoking. Remember that the tissue of the lung is the skin. Smoking will also compromise your skin quality.

4. Excessive drinking can cause liver problems. However, according to TCM, the liver has additional and very different functions than it does in Western medicine. For women, if the liver is out of balance, it will affect the stomach's function and cause menstrual cycle disorders and emotional problems. If liver problems continue, a woman might eventually experience Qi stagnation in the liver meridian. This meridian runs through the breast area. Other symptoms of liver Qi disorders include breast tenderness before periods, headaches on the sides of the head during the menstrual cycle, continual stomach bloating, bad breath, and a red nose (which is due to excess internal heat in the stomach). Men also experience these same problems. Drinking a glass of wine occasionally may not harm you, but if you want to protect your liver and healthy liver function, avoid drinking any alcoholic beverage to excess.

5. In TCM's view, sex consumes a great deal of Qi. Here is another area where you can save your Qi for healing the root cause of your excess weight. Too much sex will cause liver and kidney Qi deficiencies. If you're a woman, you might experience a lot of vaginal discharge. For both men and women, overdoing sex can cause fatigue, chronic lower back pain, insomnia, ringing in the ears, heel pain, hair loss, and even infertility. If you really overdo sex, you can even experience eye problems. Changing sex partners frequently uses up too much liver and kidney Qi and can cause additional problems. You also might contract a sexually transmitted disease if you do not protect yourself. Naturally, if you have other health problems, this can compromise any effort to self-heal and lose weight.

6. Many people have been told that they are doing the right thing by exercising vigorously. They've been told that high-impact exercise will help protect their cardiovascular health and help them lose or control weight. TCM regards exercise differently. First of all, the body is approximately 70 percent water. A water-type body needs water-type exercises to match its energy frequency. Also, TCM theory states that the tendon is the "tissue" of the liver and is governed by this organ. Tendons are like any other structures in the body: they have their limits in terms of function. In this case, a tendon is like a rubber band; you can only stretch it so many times before it loses its elasticity or ability to perform.

High-impact exercises often cause tendon problems that, in turn, can affect the liver and create a liver function disorder. In fact, some women who overexercise do not menstruate or have trouble with their periods. They have developed a liver function disorder that now impedes the free flow of Qi and blood in their body.

I see a lot of women and some men who suffer from chronic fatigue syndrome—almost all of them have a history of over-exercising, especially with high-impact aerobics. I recommend soft exercises like dancing, Yoga, Taiji, and of course noncompetitive and gentle swimming, which matches our "watery" bodies well. One of the best exercises of all is slow, gentle walking in nature, where you can tune up your body, mind, emotions, and spirit with nature's healing Qi. I recommend being fully present in nature—don't wear earphones, don't carry weights, don't speed walk. If you want to test your cardiovascular condition and go beyond the physical level, pay particular attention to the last movement in our *Wu Ming* Meridian Therapy *The Dragon Stands Between Heaven and Earth* (#10). I've challenged a lot of people to stand in this position for more than five minutes. Even if they can run for forty minutes, or stay on a treadmill for an hour, almost no one performs this Qigong movement for more than five minutes. I challenge you also. The longer you hold this posture, the more benefit you will gain, not only for your physical heart and lung, but also for your spirit.

7. If you're a frequent drug user—whether nonprescription or prescription—it's likely that your symptoms are being addressed instead of their root cause. Most drugs are constructed in such a way as to suppress a problem instead of healing its root cause. All drugs are toxic to some degree; they must all eventually be processed through your liver. For your own health, you need to identify the root cause of your problem instead of continually addressing its symptoms. Sooner or later, the health problem you believe you're treating can emerge in another part of your body. If you're under drug treatment, you can also look for complementary treatments that can help strengthen your Qi, so you might eventually be able to reduce your drug dosage. This way, your immune system can become stronger and can allow your own natural healing ability to take over. Work with your doctor to see what is possible.

8. Birth control pills affect the liver, which TCM states, is the most important organ for women's health. TCM believes that unless the liver functions in harmony with your other or-

gans, you cannot get pregnant. To help women who have difficulty getting pregnant, TCM treats the liver and coaxes it back into balance so that it functions smoothly with all the other organs. Because birth control pills suppress your ability to become pregnant, they also suppress your liver's function.

Women who have been taking birth control pills for many years often experience difficulty getting pregnant because their liver function has become impaired. Remember, here we are not referring to the physical liver. I have helped quite a few women who were infertile become pregnant. When they come to see me, they tell me that they have done all the tests possible and that their liver "is in good condition." I help them understand that while the scientific tests show their physical organ is all right, my TCM diagnosis shows that the function of their liver is definitely out of balance. When the whole body isn't working in harmony, a lot of things can go wrong.

VI. SELF-HEALING CHECKLIST FOR FREQUENT DISCOMFORTS

1. Do you suffer from PMS?
2. Do you suffer from hay fever?
3. Do you suffer physical symptoms when the weather or the seasons changes?
4. Do you frequently have bad breath?
5. Do your ears ring?
6. Are your nails brittle or cracked?
7. Is your nose area red all the time?
8. Do your eyes tear frequently?
9. Do you have frequent headaches?
10. Do you suffer from adult acne?

ANSWER SECTION ON FREQUENT DISCOMFORTS

1. There is some controversy in the West as to whether or not PMS really exists. TCM has a long history of successful

treatment of the complex of PMS symptoms, which it relates to a liver function disorder. PMS has a wide range of associated problems, such as many different types of headaches including migraines, nausea, constipation, loose stool, anger, depression, mood swings, among others. The root cause of all of these seemingly unrelated conditions is the same—liver Qi stagnation. As long as the liver function disorder remains untreated, these problems will remain. I often see patients who regard PMS as simply something they must put up with every month, uncomfortable as it is. I really try to educate these women about this condition and what a serious warning sign it is. I urge them to treat the root cause. If they don't, they are in for more health problems ahead. Almost always, women with PMS have a difficult menopause.

2. Hay fever usually occurs in the spring and fall. According to TCM, if an organ's energy function cannot match a season's energy change, then you will become sick. Spring is the season of the liver, and the eye is the "window" of the liver. If you get hay fever in the spring, you might have the most trouble with itchy, watering eyes. Fall is the season of the lung, and the nose is its "window." Accordingly, if you get hay fever in the fall, you might experience the most trouble with a runny nose. No matter what season, if your organs are out of balance with Universal energy changes, you will most likely experience some kind of health problem. Fixing the organ's function is the way to permanently address this problem; covering up the symptoms with medications is only a temporary measure.

3. If your body's Qi or energy is not in harmony when weather or seasonal changes occur, your body will produce different kinds of health problems. For example, if your body has too much dampness or maintains a lot of water, then when it's damp or the rainy season comes, you may experience arthritic pain. If you always catch a cold or the flu in the winter, the season that the kidney rules, your condition is related to a kidney Qi deficiency. If you experience headaches at the top of your head or excessive anger or mood swings when winter turns to spring, your liver function is out of balance. If you have heart problems or heart disease, you might experience a lot of discomfort in the summer, whose ruling organ is the heart. Women in transition should be extra careful during seasonal changes.

4. Bad breath is one indication that your body has liver Qi stagnation. This condition can, in turn, cause your stomach Qi to overheat. Emotional problems or stress can bring about this kind of bad breath. Look for healthy ways to relieve any emotional discomfort, especially if it is chronic. For instance, TCM has one way to reduce stress. As we've seen, you can buy a dozen eggs and smash them. Or, you can smash raw potatoes by stomping on them. Or, in a safe place, break glass bottles. Although these actions may seem a little unusual, they are time-tested TCM ways to help relieve anger. Fried, barbecued, and/or spicy foods can generate excess heat in your stomach and eventually cause a stomach function disorder. Try to avoid these foods whenever possible. Make sure you have regular bowel movements.

5. If you do not have a physical problem with your ears, ringing, or tinnitus, means you have a kidney Qi deficiency. You should regard this as a serious health sign because, according to TCM, the kidney is the foundation of the body's overall Qi.

There are certain foods you can add to your diet to help increase kidney Qi. Eat any kind of seafood, including shrimp, lobsters, clams, oysters, salmon, tuna, etc. You can also add black beans, walnuts, and other nuts as often as possible. When this condition persists, TCM treats it with herbs or acupuncture.

6. TCM believes that you can identify internal health conditions by examining external physical signs. For instance, your nails are the mirrors of your liver. If your liver is healthy, your nails should be shiny, grow fast, and not break easily. If your nails are in poor condition and crack or break easily, your liver function is out of balance and you must treat it. Gelatin, shellfish, and clams can help your nails improve. Examine your nails periodically; if the half moons are not white and full, your liver Qi is weakening or becoming deficient. Take care of yourself, because this is an early warning sign of internal imbalances.

7. In TCM theory, if the nose area is red, then the stomach is suffering from excess heat. This condition is also sometimes related to unbalanced liver function. Unless the condition is fixed from the inside out, most treatments are temporary. Acupuncture, herbs, and lifestyle changes can help alleviate this condition.

8. The Five Element Theory tells us that the eyes are the "window" of the liver. If your eyes tear frequently, or if you wake up with matter in your eyes, your liver Qi is stagnating. A liver Qi dysfunction has now progressed to a physical problem. It is important to treat the root cause of this condition before it progresses further and reaches more advanced stages. Acupuncture, herbs, and lifestyle changes can also make a beneficial difference.

9. According to TCM theory, the meridians of six different organs run through the head. Qi stagnation in one or a combination of these meridians can theoretically cause 720 different kinds of headaches ($6 \times 5 \times 4 \times 3 \times 2 \times 1 = 720$). To treat a headache effectively, it is essential to identify which organ (or organs) is out of balance. For instance, headaches on both sides of the head relate to the gallbladder; headaches at the front of the head relate to the stomach, and headaches at the top of the head are associated with the liver and kidney.

Taking painkillers may temporarily alleviate headaches, but they can mask more serious problems which can emerge later. As you can see, headaches are merely symptoms telling you that there is a deeper problem, which resides in one or more of your five major organs. You can also see that headaches are specific to the individual. A man's headache may be different from his wife's, as yours may be different from your mother's. That is why pain relievers only work for some people some of the time.

10. If you suffer from adult acne, TCM theory states that your liver and kidney organs are out of balance and not functioning in harmony. The messages that they need to exchange to keep your skin clear and unblemished are not being communicated properly. Unless you restore balance in this important relationship, it is unlikely that your acne will improve permanently with topical treatments. TCM believes that it is essential to treat adult acne from the inside out. Chronic anger and stress are two of the major causes of this condition.

All of these checklists are based on the principles and theories of TCM. You may find some of the answers surprising. If you've answered yes to many of them, I urge you to be careful. Your lifestyle is directly related to your weight problems. Making changes, particularly in areas where you are under significant and or continual stress, can make a very big difference in your success with The Dragon's Way. I would like you to remember that stress is the true villain when it comes to issues of weight. Do not be fooled by focusing on food. Stress, as well as anger, overthinking and anxiety, is the Qi-stopping factor that causes everything in your body to become sluggish and pile on the pounds. Take some quiet time with yourself to reflect on the many ways stress and these other emotions affect you throughout your day. Just notice them. Do not berate yourself for being under stress; you are definitely not alone. Now, gently remind yourself that you will look for as many ways as you can to reduce or eliminate the stress, overthinking or worry that threatens to unbalance you. Every time you succeed, congratulate and acknowledge yourself for taking a positive step toward health and healing. Now, let's move on to the next stage of The Dragon's Way.

CHAPTER 5

THE PREPARATION WEEK AND WEEK 1:
Getting Your Mind and Body Ready for the Special Journey Ahead

PREPARATION WEEK

Most people understand the process of "ready, set, go." That's how I like to think about the preparation week. You are not exactly starting The Dragon's Way, but you are getting ready. What should you do? Buy a notebook in which you can keep a Healing Journal. You can use this to jot down different thoughts, observations, etc. You might even find yourself making small drawings and the like. Use it to express yourself and your feelings. Often, people are amazed when they look back at the many layers and levels of transformation that they've gone through as a result of The Dragon's Way. Go to your TCM Self-Healing Tool Box. Review the Eating for Healing foods and recipes, shop for the foods that you'll need, read over the instructions for the *Wu Ming* Meridian Qigong movements in Chapter 3. Then relax and rest. I really mean this. Try to get at least seven or eight hours of sleep each night. If you can, try and take a nap during the day.

Find some time to do nothing. If it's at night, look at the night sky and the stars. If it's during the day, try to take a slow walk in a park. Really rest and relax.

I tell all my students and participants to eat their favorite foods at what I call the "Last Meal." I urge you also to do this because after the program you may never want to eat these foods again, or at least not in the same way you do now. When your body changes, tastes for certain foods can change as well. As your body heals itself, you will be most surprised at what it chooses to like and dislike. There is no right or wrong way to heal. You are unique and you will heal in a unique way.

In this preparation week, gradually eliminate meat, fowl, fish, and cheese from your meals. This will prepare your body for the weeks ahead. Remember that these particular foods put too much of a burden on your body to digest them. This is Qi you can start to conserve immediately for self-healing!

There is one other thing that you should begin this week. This will stimulate your energy foundation. Learn *The Dragon Stands Between Heaven and Earth* (#10); it is the last movement in *Wu Ming* Meridian Therapy Qigong. It is easy to learn. Practice it every day that you can for as long as you can.

WEEK 1

Start this journey with an open mind and an open heart. Tell yourself that, at last, you're doing something about the root cause of your excess weight. And, congratulate yourself for having the intuition to have been drawn to information that can, once and for all, deal with this issue.

In Week 1, you will begin to prepare your body for deeper healing. You've already cut out meat, fowl, fish, and dairy. You should feel a little lighter now. Now you will eliminate raw vegetables and salads, bread, pasta and other carbohydrates from your daily diet. Again, I want you to be clear about why we are doing this. Your body uses up extra Qi to process these foods. During these six weeks, I want you to save every bit of excess Qi we can find to help your body heal itself. We are not making these foods "bad." The more you can avoid them, the more healing power you can draw on to correct the underlying root cause of your excess weight.

Learn the first five *Wu Ming* Meridian Therapy Qigong movements in the previous chapter and start practicing them daily. *These ancient Qigong movements are the most important part of The Dragon's Way.* Although the foods for healing are very important, as is reducing stress, it is the practice of these movements that can propel Qi, or life force, through your body to help it rebalance itself and work in harmony, the way it was meant to do. This is one of the fundamental differences between The Dragon's Way and other weight loss programs you may have tried. I believe that not one of them addressed the underlying root cause of your excess weight or helped increase your healing ability. Virtually all Western weight loss programs and products work at the material level; none can reach beyond this to the Qi or energy level like The Dragon's Way.

To begin to understand the value of this program and its ancient wisdom more fully, you will learn about two fundamental TCM theories that have been in place for more than five thousand years: Qi and Blood and the Theory of Yin and Yang.

The first week of The Dragon's Way is a time to get yourself and your body ready for the weeks to come. The learning curve during this week is exciting. Congratulate yourself. At last, with this six-week course, you are finally addressing the root cause of your weight problems. I recommend that you take things slowly at this time so you don't feel overwhelmed. Always remember to be good to yourself. Don't push things. Don't stress yourself out over this program. Remember what stress can do to your body. Be happy that fate has helped you choose a book that can offer a real time-tested solution to your weight condition. (And by time-tested, we don't mean it was invented in the last year, or the last decade, or even the last century.) You're on your way—you are on The Dragon's Way!

SOME THINGS TO THINK ABOUT DURING WEEK 1

As you open the door to The Dragon's Way, let me remind you again that the real purpose of the program is to help you learn how to take care of yourself and become healthier and that losing weight and inches will be a byproduct of this effort. Our Dragon's Way program has helped close to a thousand people get just to where you really want to be. Healthy—with less weight and fewer inches.

Remember, some people lose more inches than pounds at first. The weight will come off, but for some it can take time, depending on the desired amount of pounds you want to shed and the state of your health when you begin. Everyone starts at their own level. There is no competition. But even if you don't see immediate results, healing is happening, and this is the real difference of The Dragon's Way. Things are changing underneath. It must, because Qigong is all about helping to strengthen your Qi so that your body begins to function properly. When that happens, weight starts to drop off naturally. It's like the approach of spring. Although it may not be readily apparent, beneath the surface, nature is working hard to push out the buds that will bloom into magnificent flowers, or make the sap rise in trees so that leaves will bud. The same is true for some of you reading this book. It doesn't happen overnight. Don't let anyone fool you. When it comes to *healthy* weight loss, there are no "quick fixes." There are many ways to lose weight—but none that can address the root cause from an ancient holistic medical theory framework. That's where The Dragon's Way is unique.

We've already talked about the concept of "losing" weight. Rather than looking at getting rid of excess weight as a "loss," it's better to think of this process as "taking off," "giving up," "shedding," or "eliminating" something you no longer need. Your excess weight is not a loss because you definitely don't want it back! In fact, you undoubtedly would be happy if you never saw it again. Now you're beginning to think like a Taoist, one who follows the Way of the Tao, not a religion, but a philosophical way of being and looking at the world. You'll come to learn that your thoughts are very powerful and that they do indeed create your reality. I urge you to begin thinking about, well . . . about thinking. Choose your thoughts carefully because they help you create your own world. What kind of world would you like?

Beginning with this first week of The Dragon's Way, I'd also like you to pay attention to the way you choose food in the supermarket and how you feel about the food you put into your mouth. For example, are you selecting something at the store because it captures your eye or because you think you *should* have it? Are you choosing foods subconsciously or unconsciously? When you eat, take notice of what it tastes like. Is it satisfying? Does it taste fresh to you? Are you eating because you're hungry, because you think you're hungry, or are you doing it for other reasons? If you've started your journal and want to keep a diary of your initial thoughts and observations, then begin this week. Just use this information to gain insight, do not let it rule your life. You may have some interesting things to tell yourself.

During this time, I'd also like you to recognize how brave you are for walking down this unfamiliar path. But let me assure you that these six weeks offer you a great adventure if you are willing to "go with the flow," a very important TCM concept.

In your life's journey, there are so many directions from which you can choose. You can choose the familiar. As an analogy, think of your life as a car trip that you have planned for a long time. You can set off on a course that lets you take the interstate highways; these are well-recognized roads and these will definitely get you to your destination faster. Or, you can decide to take a more interesting route that takes you along some scenic local roads that you might never have experienced had you not taken the time to plan this very special journey. This way lies more excitement and more of the unknown. Away from the monotonous, predictable hum of the interstate, you might find interesting people, family stores, terrific little restaurants, drive-in movies, and other unexpected possibilities. If you're unmarried, you might even stop and find the person of your dreams!

I believe that for people in Western cultures, TCM can represent the local route I've just described. You see, by approaching The Dragon's Way with curiosity, optimism, and enthusiasm, your whole life can start to change. It can become richer, healthier, and more fun than you ever imagined. Nothing about The Dragon's Way is meant to be tedious or meant to deprive you of happiness. In fact, I tell my own participants, "I don't want to take away anything that you love. Your love is stronger than my program. Be happy and do your best. When you are happy, you can change."

One other thing to think about: TCM looks at medicine as an art, and the true source of that art is Qi (pronounced *chee*), or vital energy. Therefore, those who practice this medicine are considered to be like any real artist. You are either born with this "gift" or not. A good Chinese doctor knows this is true. Therefore, he or she regards the various healing methods as vehicles to transfer his or her gift of healing to the person who is ill or unbalanced. To do so, TCM texts say, it is the doctor's task to choose the best treatment, and likewise it is the patient's responsibility to be a good partner and an open and willing recipient of care. If this mutually respectful relationship is not in place, it is difficult to achieve the best results.

A good TCM practitioner understands that you must treat the whole person, but he or she can also save Qi by connecting with the patient's own Qi and helping the patient jumpstart it; otherwise, the practitioner needs to spend his or her own Qi to help the patient. In car analogy terms, in the former case, the doctor has to take the battery out of the car and replace it, or tow it to a garage where this can happen; in the latter, the doctor just provides a good energy boost.

Highly skilled TCM practitioners understand that the patient's own body is ten times more powerful and its energy field ten times greater than the doctor's. If your own Qi can be sparked, then your body will begin to do the job of healing. Also, if you can help yourself heal, you will be able to draw on, and build on, that skill to help yourself prevent future problems. Remember, The Dragon's Way is also about giving you the healing tools you need for the rest of your life.

THE ANCIENT ENERGY MOVEMENTS: *WU MING* QIGONG

I'd like to give you a deeper understanding about the most essential part of The Dragon's Way, the *Wu Ming* Meridian Therapy Qigong movements, the series of ancient energy movements that powers this program. The *Wu Ming* Qigong system, which works for self-healing and increasing internal Qi, descends directly from the ancient Taoist masters Lao Tzu (sixth century B.C.) and Chuang Tzu (fourth century B.C.). Its secrets have been passed down from one master to another for many, many centuries. In China, there are thousands of Qigong forms; some are very ancient like *Wu Ming*, others are modern systems created by modern masters. Our Qigong school is the only one in the United States that teaches this ancient form of Qigong. And our educational healing programs are the only ones based on this form.

I call Qigong a "practice." TCM has understood its efficacy for millennia as one of the most remarkable and powerful healing systems that can benefit people of all ages. It is actually the most important and powerful healing tool I can share with you. I want you to know that I also "practice" every spare moment

I have. Without continual practice, it would be difficult for me to provide high-quality healing benefit to my patients. I am also very lucky because, in my life, fate has given me a number of masters. To each of them I am very grateful for the special "keys of understanding" that have been passed to me, or I inherited, from their powerful lineages. These healing secrets have helped make my TCM practice unique. Now, it is part of my mission to share this special information with as many people as possible.

QIGONG PRACTICE

Now refer back to Chapter 3 and review the instructions for the *Wu Ming* Meridian Therapy. I recommend reading the instructions and studying the photos for all ten Qigong movements—then go back and concentrate on learning and practicing the first five. They are simple movements that virtually anyone can do almost anywhere. They require no equipment other than an open heart and, if you can do it, an empty mind.

Familiarize yourself with each of the five movements. Try them out to see how they feel. Now, slow each movement down. These are not aerobic in nature. They are designed to help relieve Qi stagnation in your meridians—the invisible energy pathways that run through your body and connect its structures. These are slow, gentle "meridian stretches" that can stimulate your Qi and get it flowing through your meridians and your organs so that your body begins to work in harmony again as it was meant to do. As you practice, you will begin to experience how good it feels to stretch your meridians slowly and gently. You may also feel the Qi or energy beginning to flow more freely again throughout your body. Practicing daily can definitely bring you many healing benefits.

During Week 1, here are the four new Qigong movements you should learn and practice. Look back in Chapter 3 for descriptions of how to practice these movements. Continue to practice #10 and increase the amount of time you can hold this posture:

Number 1: The Dragon's Toe Dance
Number 2: The Dragon Kicks Forward
Number 3: The Dragon's Twist
Number 4: The Dragon's Punch
Number 10: The Dragon Stands Between Heaven and Earth

Number 10 is a most important posture. This is something you can do daily for the rest of your life. Maximum healing can be gained from practicing the entire set of movements in the morning and again, at night, for twenty minutes each session. If you can only practice once a day, that's all right. It is a quality twenty-minute practice that we're after, not quantity. If you want to see benefits more quickly, then besides a quality practice, you should practice these movements as frequently and as long as possible.

If you practice regularly throughout The Dragon's Way, you will definitely establish a new and healthy habit, one that you will feel good about continuing (I hope for the rest of your life!). Why? Because you will feel so much better and more alive when you practice. On Day 1 of Week 1, it may be hard for you to imagine, but you'll find that practicing *Wu Ming* Meridian Therapy will soon become a welcome, important part of your day, as essential as your daily shower.

I think that this story is one of many that illustrates how life-changing going to the root cause of excess weight can be.

Ten years ago when I was twenty-six, I lost 120 pounds with a popular diet program. In spite of my best efforts to keep it off, the weight crept back on. I tried a variety of plans and prescription medications. All of them were somewhat successful, but only in the short term. When I found

*The Dragon's Way, I had not only regained 130 pounds,
but now had a number of physical symptoms that totally
exhausted me. I was caught in a vicious cycle, which pre-
vented me from handling the challenges of being a wife,
mother of two, and administrative assistant in an advertising agency. I began practicing* Wu Ming *Meridian Therapy daily. I began to understand how it was possible for
me to awaken my healing abilities. What hope it gave me!
So far, I've lost about twenty-three pounds, but my menstrual cycle is regular again, my digestion has improved,
and my energy has soared. Now, I think about health, not
about weight. It's a pleasure to shop for foods that heal,
and I find I spend less money. I am so grateful to The
Dragon's Way for helping me get control of my life and
my health.*

SHELLEY E., 36-YEAR-OLD ADMINISTRATIVE ASSISTANT

Once again I want to emphasize that The Dragon's Way
Qigong movements are gentle and relaxing. They are *not* exercises to develop muscles or physical strength (although more
physical strength will come from them). They are designed to
help relieve hunger, stimulate your own healing ability and increase your Qi. It is only through continued practice of these
simple movements that you will be able to experience the benefits they offer. If you do, they will infuse you with Qi and begin
to heal the root cause of your weight problem. Here, once and
for all, you're finally dealing with the fundamental conditions
that produce excess weight. Feel the relief in that thought! You
can do this. How do I know? Because close to one thousand
people have been happy and satisfied with their Dragon's Way
experience. We think you will too.

*I must have lost and gained more than sixty-five pounds
more than once. I think now I have finally learned how to
take care of myself so that when I lose all the weight, it won't*

*come back on. I know now that my weight is only one symp-
tom of my body's out-of-balance state. I had a lot of other
uncomfortable symptoms such as fatigue, back pain, muscle
tension, headaches, insomnia, depression, worry, frequent urination, palpitations and forgetfulness. I say "had" because
almost all of them are gone along with about sixteen pounds.
I know I have more weight to take off, and this time I feel
confident the extra pounds are going for good. I really liked
the meridian therapy and knowing that I was balancing my
organs with it and how I ate. Hunger wasn't a problem. In
fact, my appetite reduced without doing anything. I think
that it was getting balanced too. I think self-healing is the
self-balancing that happens when we give our bodies what
they need.*

SHARON N., 42-YEAR-OLD SYSTEMS ANALYST

EATING FOR HEALING

This week you will also begin to think about food consumption in a different way. Rather than eating simply to eat, I'd
like for you to begin thinking about food in terms of its healing energy. Please don't take these thoughts as another way
to add more stress in your life. I recommend that you just
start to listen and respond to the true messages of your body
when selecting certain foods to eat. You might be surprised
at what you learn.

During this first week, eat the foods that you like at one
meal, especially those that are your particular favorites. Eat a
lot of them. Why do I tell my Dragon's Way people to do this?
They think they have the answer. "Because we'll be giving them
up for six weeks and we'll want to eat them, but we shouldn't,"
was one response—albeit an incorrect one. The real reason I
want you to eat all the foods that you like today is that there's
a good chance you simply won't be interested in them after The

Dragon's Way. One woman in class was incredulous. "Oh come on, how could I not love my pint of Ben & Jerry's Cookie Dough Ice Cream?" Another said, "I can't ever see me really giving up pasta. It's a way of life for me. Besides, I'm Italian!"

Well, as I tell The Dragon's Way students, it's not that you'll hate these foods, but you'll be more than satisfied with just a bite or two of them. Or, you may be somewhat indifferent to them. They won't have the same hold on you that they used to. You'll be able to take them or leave them, depending on how your body feels. It's amazing how many people at the conclusion of our program have no interest or taste for their old favorites. So I recommend you eat all your favorite foods now!

Throughout The Dragon's Way, you will eat breakfast, lunch and dinner. It is essential to eat meals at regular times. Again, just like a car, you've got to have enough fuel to get where you're going. Don't fool yourself: a healthy body needs enough food for the stomach and spleen to do their job of transforming the foods you eat into what TCM called nutritive essence. You need this to keep all of your body's functions running in top order.

TCM's point of view on breakfast is that it is a very important meal that should not be missed. Morning is when it's best to eat the *richest* foods of your day. When you wake up, your stomach is empty. Your body has rested throughout the night and needs Qi to get going and to power itself for the tasks of the day, and therefore should be given good, high-quality food. Don't try to tough it out in the morning with no food, then at 10:30 or 11:00 A.M. eat a bagel or a donut and a cup of coffee. Or, worse yet, have a cigarette. Where do you think the Qi to run your body comes from when you haven't given it fuel? It steals Qi from your kidney, an organ you'll soon discover is vital to your very life span, not to mention the proper regulation of water in your lower body.

In the afternoon, when you eat lunch, it should be your *biggest* meal of the day. Dinner, on the other hand, should be your smallest. Eating a big meal late at night interrupts your ability to sleep well. This is when your digestive system needs its natural rest. Your body's Qi should not be working throughout the night to power the digestive function; instead it should be peacefully sleeping and recharging itself. Remember, in The Dragon's Way, one of our goals is to continually look out for opportunities to conserve Qi so that it can be applied to alleviating the presenting symptom of excess weight.

Unfortunately, I see many patients who eat their biggest meal late at night. If you're one of those people who always eats a big meal, then goes to sleep, you are forcing your stomach to work overtime all night long just to digest this meal. This can really disrupt your sleep, even causing disturbing dreams or uncomfortable heartburn. Ideally, to keep your body in balance, when you wake up, the food you had the day before should be fully digested and you should be on "empty." That's the ideal way a healthy body starts its new day. As you can see, eating a lighter meal at night can help conserve a lot of Qi.

If you have not already done so, I would like you to eliminate, as much as possible, meat, fowl, fish, cheese, and any beans from your meals this week. Eliminating sources of excess protein from your meals will help you do two things: cleanse your body and save more Qi for the purpose of revitalizing your organ system. This enables it to function again. In other words, your organs need a break! Trust the program and try to eliminate these foods now.

People in the West are conditioned to think that eating less food is not a good thing, but eating less, if done properly and balanced with a practice like Qigong, is actually a very effective healing practice. Think about people who go away for a special supervised week of fasting. Many return happy, rejuvenated, and feeling better than they ever did.

When people first start The Dragon's Way, many are convinced they can't possibly get through it without eating their favorite high-protein meal or protein food supplement. Let me assure you that it is *very* possible and not even that difficult. There's actually plenty of protein-rich food to eat within The Dragon's Way without depending on these sources of protein for the next six weeks. Believe it or not, walnuts or pine nuts are excellent foods, and I recommend that you include them with breakfast each morning. The walnuts and fruit are suggested to give you a really solid Qi foundation and a good amount of quality energy to begin your day. Also remember, you are building up your Qi by practicing Qigong daily.

Trust the program and help your Qi stop working overtime Give your body this six-week break to really begin to heal. The results will speak for themselves. You will be amazed at how well and energized you feel. Our Eating for Healing plan only works in a healthy way in conjunction with The Dragon's Way movements. You could use the plan without the movements, but it would take you much longer to heal the root cause of your weight problem. And, I believe, without the Qigong to strengthen your body and help the organs work in harmony again, any weight loss could be temporary.

The list of Recommended Energy Healing Foods is in Chapter 2. Add as many of the foods from this list as possible into your daily diet and eat according to the meal suggestions. While it is all right to eat other vegetables and fruits, try to stick to the recommended foods as closely as possible. I have chosen these foods specifically for their ability to help heal three organs that are most frequently out of balance with people in Western society who have weight problems: the kidney, liver, and spleen. I've also chosen them for their ability to help your body eliminate water, fat, and toxins. Each of these foods knows exactly which organ it should heal and is sent there by the lung. That's right. It's the lung's job to distribute the nutritive essence that gets made by your stomach and spleen organ partnership. (Now, you might wonder how is the lung involved in weight issues? Please read on and you will see how *all* the five major organs— lung, heart, spleen, liver, and kidney—must work together in harmony to keep your body functioning well and your weight under control.)

These everyday foods will be gentle on your body and will not use up a great deal of your Qi to digest. This is another way to "bank" extra Qi to help your organs come back into harmony again and work as one complete well-oiled machine, so to speak. To add variety to this Eating for Healing Plan, we've created more than forty recipes in Chapter 12 that are made up from the foods on the list. If you like to cook, go ahead and be creative on your own! Use these foods in whatever combinations you like.

During this first week, I'd also like you to gradually stop eating heavy carbohydrates—potatoes, grains, and all their products such as bread, couscous, etc. Although you can have a half-cup of pasta or rice if you feel you need it. Also, please begin to change your habits and eliminate cold drinks as well as cold and raw foods, including salads. Switch to warm liquids whenever possible and if you eat raw vegetables, cook them lightly before eating. You can dip them in boiling water for a few minutes to take the chill off of them.

I know that some of you are thinking that cooking vegetables destroys or reduces their nutrient content. However, when they are not cooked, your stomach finds them hard to digest, because their essence is cold. The nature of the stomach is warmth-loving. You may not know it, but your organs must operate within nature's law. Your stomach really doesn't like cold things, especially if it's fed a continuous diet of cold foods. If you're eating this way, you're literally going against the nature of your stomach. What happens when you do this? Eventually you can get sick, or at the very least you can trip up the way your stomach functions. Why is that so important? The stomach has relationships with a number of other organs that can also become unbalanced as well, causing—you're correct, weight gain. The result? Weight that you simply cannot lose, no matter how hard you try. Why? Because the underlying root problem of an organ function disorder has not been addressed, let alone fixed.

During the time you have committed to study and participate in The Dragon's Way, you will gain the greatest healing benefit from your foods if they are cooked. It doesn't matter how long you cook the vegetables; their healing essence is still there. However, most people find that cooking vegetables to the point where they are still slightly crunchy and reach a bright color is sufficient and the most enjoyable. From a healing perspective, I sincerely encourage you to cater to your stomach's natural preferences. The rewards for making this simple, easy change are great.

Now, let's talk about water. Usually in my first class there are a few people who invariably bring their "water bottle" with them. These are the people who are very surprised when we discuss the TCM point of view about water. If you're accustomed to drinking a lot of water every day, I must tell you, in your best interest, please stop. You're probably drinking when you're not even thirsty because you've heard through a weight loss program or plan, or fashion and fitness article, that it's a good idea to drink before meals to cut down on your appetite. Or, you've always heard that drinking eight glasses of water a day is good for you, that it will flush out toxins. Lots of health magazines talk about hydration as a healthy practice.

The TCM truth? For most people, drinking eight glasses of water a day is way too much water! Start to seriously listen to your body—not your mind. When your body feels thirsty, then drink something. If you find that you are genuinely thirsty all of the time, then you might be one of those people who have a problem of too much internal heat. In this case, you can benefit not by drinking water, but by drinking watermelon juice, a Dragon's Way top healing food. TCM practitioners have prescribed watermelon for centuries because its healing essence has the ability to cool down conditions of internal heat and relieve the body of toxins.

Here's The Dragon's Way to look at water consumption. I often ask our program participants if, when they go to sleep at night, they leave their car's engine running outside in their driveway. No, of course they don't. They shut off their automobile's engine and turn it on again when they're ready to go somewhere. If you drink too much water, your body is constantly running its Qi or energy—even through the night—your kidney and your bladder are constantly in a state of production, when, in fact, they should be resting and conserving Qi—the very Qi you need to heal the imbalances of weight problems! I recommend that you drink only when you feel you *need* water. And then I strongly recommend that you drink cool or room temperature water. Your stomach literally "hates" to receive cold things. (Even the ice cream that tastes so good in your mouth makes your stomach wince.) I am not telling you to give up ice cream and other cold foods. What TCM is telling you is that when your body is truly healed, you'll be able to pretty much eat whatever you like, without gaining weight, if you follow the principles of The Dragon's Way. This is a gift that can last you a lifetime.

Just switching to warm foods, room temperature liquids, and selecting foods with a warm essence like ginger, cinnamon, fennel, and clove can make a big difference in the way you feel. I urge you to follow these guidelines for just these six weeks. I think you'll be amazed at the results. If you suffer from stomach problems like bloating, stomachaches, burping, gas, and the like, you should also see a marked improvement as you progress through this program.

TCM LESSON OF THE WEEK

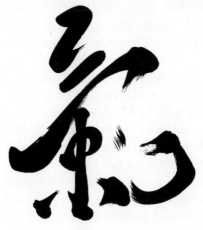

The Theory of Qi: How It Works in Your Energy Savings and Checking Accounts

As we discussed in the introduction, TCM has been practiced continuously for more than five thousand years. What is known is that TCM's true origins occurred long before its principles and theories were written down twenty-five hundred years ago in the *Huang Di Nei Jing* (pronounced *whong dee nay jeeng*), considered to be the first TCM medical "textbook." This comprehensive work outlines the entire structure of TCM and how it should be practiced. Among many things, it describes in sharp detail—without the aid of x-rays or magnetic resonance imaging (MRI)—the human body and how it works. The *Nei Jing* reveals a great deal about Qi. We learn from this early text that we have two different kinds of Qi: Inborn and Acquired. To better help our Dragon's Way participants and you understand this concept, I've borrowed an almost ideal analogy from Western banking practices. I call Inborn Qi our savings account and Acquired Qi our checking account.

Simply put, Inborn Qi is the energy foundation that we inherit from our parents. This kind of Qi is stored in the kidney.

Its quantity and quality are determined by the quantity and quality of your mother's and father's Qi, the kind of pregnancy your mother had, and the time, place, and nature of your birth. This particular Qi or energy foundation cannot be changed. Most important, you have received a finite supply. When it's completely used up, it's time to die. When my patients ask me, "How much Inborn Qi do I have?," I tell them it is up to fate, but what you do with it, how you spend it, and how well you take care of it are your responsibility. The *Nei Jing* tells us: "Your life belongs to God (or the Universe); your health belongs to you."

Ancient Chinese texts also tell us that Inborn Qi determines your basic constitution—both physical and mental—and governs your growth and development. If you have had children or had the opportunity to watch young children grow, you know what I am talking about. We often see that problems with Qi can be passed on to a child if, during a woman's pregnancy, her nutrition is poor or she is sick. For example, a baby born without strong Qi might have a soft spot on top of the head that closes later than normal; a toddler might take longer to stand up because he or she doesn't have enough strength in the knees; or a child's dental development might be delayed. All of these problems are related to the bone, and in TCM, all matters related to the bone are controlled by the kidney—the storehouse of Inborn Qi. When working with babies and children who have bone problems, I always treat their kidney with an herb tonic or bone soup to strengthen this organ.

TCM also says that the quantity and quality of Inborn Qi also determines how long we live. Even though TCM believes this is true, insightful practitioners also recognize that how we manage our allotted Qi and the time we've been given is up to each of us. I believe that everyone has a mission. The nature of your mission may not be readily accessible to you on a conscious level, but when your mission is accomplished, it's time to leave this earthly plane. Unfortunately for many of us, we rely far too heavily on and draw far too frequently on our savings account of Inborn Qi; we use its precious "funds" wastefully. When we've emptied this account, it's time to die.

Luckily, the *Nei Jing* describes another readily available source from which we can withdraw energy: Acquired Qi, or our checking account, which is stored in our spleen/stomach organ system. Acquired Qi supports the function of all the organs, and helps maintain the body's ability to regulate and heal itself. The good part about this checking account of Acquired Qi is that unlike our savings account, we can actually add Qi or vital energy to it. How? By eating high-quality foods in the proper amounts at the proper times; by ensuring that our organs are functioning well; by practicing energy-saving Qigong movements; and by learning how to manage Qi. Thus, our personal checking account is dynamic and allows Qi to automatically and constantly flow in and move out. Through the generation and management of Acquired Qi, we have the chance to maximize the power and harmonious functioning of our body's entire system.

Unfortunately, most people don't build up enough Acquired Qi in their checking accounts and must routinely withdraw "funds" from their savings account of Inborn Qi for the day-to-day energy expenditures of life's activities. What are these activities? They include respiration, metabolism, healing from internal and external assaults, sleeping, eating, digestion, elimination, thinking, feeling, intuition, working, dealing with stress, balancing emotions, and more! This is particularly true for anyone coping with the demands of today's world and who is constantly on the go, mentally, physically, and even emotionally.

Learning how to build and strengthen your Acquired Qi is one of the most important parts of The Dragon's Way. These linked checking and savings accounts are a lifetime package deal. TCM understands that the human body does not work in any other way. Its operating rules are related to natural, not manmade law, which is quite specific and cannot be changed.

You can begin to appreciate why it's so important to build up your checking account continuously and be extremely cautious about drawing on your irreplaceable savings account of Qi. One well-known ancient Chinese doctor described this relationship in a different way: "Your life is like a candle—you can be born with a small candle or a tall candle. You have no choice in this. How you protect its flame is now up to you. If you've been given a long candle and you burn it carelessly, you will not last as long as a shorter candle that protects its flame. The better you protect your light, the longer it remains lit."

The Magnificent Dance of Yin and Yang Energies

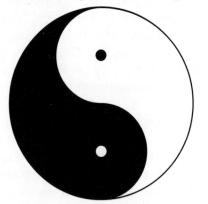

To appreciate the complexity of your body and how all its parts are integrated into one interrelated system, it's essential to understand the Theory of Yin (*eeen*) and Yang (*yahn*), as well as The Five Element Theory. TCM believes everything is composed of two complementary energies; one energy is yin and the other is yang. They are never separate; one cannot exist without the other. TCM defines this as The Yin and Yang Theory of opposition and interdependence. This intertwined and inseparable relationship is reflected in the circular yin/yang symbol seen above. Look carefully at this symbol; no matter how you divide this circle, the divided section always contains both energies—even if it is just one small dot. They are indivisible and inseparable.

Yin and yang are also part of the natural law. Age-old TCM texts say that, "If you understand yin and yang, you can hold the entire Universe in your hands." These two universal energies are in everything, including our bodies. Everything can be divided into yin and yang. Here are some examples:

YIN	YANG
Female	Male
Water	Fire
Cold	Hot
Interior	Exterior
Slow	Fast
Contraction	Expansion
Passive	Active
Deficiency	Excess
Moon	Sun
Night	Day

Everything in the body is controlled by yin and yang energies. For example, the front of your body is yin; the back of your body is yang. Your head is yang; your feet are yin. The outside of your arms and legs are yang; the inside is yin. Inside your body, Qi is considered yang; blood and body fluids are yin. The five major organs or viscera (liver, heart, spleen, lung, kidney) are yin; their respective partner organs (gallbladder, small intestine, stomach, large intestine, and bladder—called bowels in TCM) are yang.

Because yin and yang have an inseparable relationship, you can see that if you have a problem with one, the other will also. If your gallbladder suffers from an imbalance, sooner or later, it will affect your liver, its corresponding partner. The reverse is also true. It's also important to understand that despite their specific yin/yang designation, each of the organs listed above also have yin and yang energies within themselves, and these energies must also remain in harmony. When you consider these fundamental energies and the job of balancing them, and keeping them in harmony as well, you can begin to appreciate the amazingly complex, yet delicate, task of keeping these dynamic systems in equilibrium for your body, mind and spirit to remain well! You are a whole magnificent integrated and interrelated system, not just individual parts.

Why does TCM consider this theory so important to good health and weight management? Western medicine tends to look at your numbers: your blood pressure, your cholesterol numbers, your fat measure, your heart rate, among others. If your numbers are good, you are pronounced healthy. You may not feel healthy, but the numbers appear to indicate you are healthy. TCM sees you as an infinite number of relationships that must be calibrated with care not just in balance, but in harmony. Balance and harmony are important concepts. Often people think they're the same, but they are not. Balance is a manual exchange. We can place two weights on a scale and see if they balance. Harmony, on the other hand, is a more fluid state in which exchanges between things, for instance Qi and Blood, is automatic. It happens effortlessly. When a TCM practitioner perceives that your body's systems are in a state of harmony, he or she knows you are healthy. More to the point, *you* know you are healthy. No one has to tell you that you are. Conversely, no one really needs to tell you when you feel ill. Whether you have a scientific test to "prove" how you feel, your own body constantly tells you how you feel—if you'll only listen.

Let's look at another car analogy: You can own a brand new car, but if you've bought a "lemon," it just won't function properly. Your neighbor can own a ten-year-old car, and because he's maintained it lovingly over the past decade, it still runs quite well. Maybe it's not as fast as it used to be, but it's reliable, it's solid, and it never breaks down. It's the same way with individuals as they age. Older people can live healthy lives when the relationships of their organs are balanced and their yin and yang energies are in harmony. Even if they cannot perform strenuous physical activities, they eat well, they sleep well, their emotions are balanced, they are always happy, and they don't need to take an endless array of medications. For their age, they are in a state of excellent health.

You can contrast this with people who are much younger. They may suffer from indigestion problems, run themselves ragged every day, work sixty hours or more a week, and suffer from depression. They also may take large quantities of over-the-counter medications, or even drugs. Who is healthy and who is balanced? When you begin to grasp these concepts, you can see how your body really works and why certain things that we do in the West that we believe keep us healthy are really detrimental to our well-being and our weight.

Yin　　　　　　　　Yang

TCM has an ancient saying: "As long as you know the theory of yin and yang, you can be a good TCM doctor." The Qi of yin and yang are the basis of the most fundamental method of

TCM diagnosis. For instance, if I start by diagnosing a condition from the point of view of yin and yang, I can already achieve a 50 percent chance of being correct. Its root cause is either one or the other. The problem might be a yin Qi or energy problem, or it might be related to unbalanced yang Qi. Now, I can continue to improve the degree of correctness of my diagnosis and therefore treatment. Here I move on to take into consideration the other syndromes which I describe later in this book. Suffice it to say that yin/yang is extremely valuable in diagnosing and treating patients. It is particularly important to weight problems where imbalances between organ systems have caused the body to stop functioning well and stubbornly to hold onto extra pounds.

MY THOUGHTS FOR YOU THIS WEEK

This week you are starting a new adventure. You are choosing to approach your life from a different vantage point. You are doing many things that are different and this takes a lot of courage. It is not always easy to do things that are unfamiliar and perhaps a little uncomfortable. Acknowledge yourself for your willingness to make these changes in your life. I can tell you with a great deal of certainty that you will be happy that you chose The Dragon's Way.

Most of all, be kind to yourself. Try to identify the times and places in your life where you can take a few moments out to become peaceful each day. They are there for you. You just have to capture them. From now on, I encourage you to search for these healing minutes and incorporate them into your life. In these calm periods during your day or evening, you may want to write your thoughts and feelings in your Healing Journal. Have a good week and above all treat yourself well. You are a very special person!

• •

WEEK 1: FOLLOW THE STEPS OF THE DRAGON'S WAY TO HEAL THE ROOT CAUSE OF EXCESS WEIGHT

- How many times and how much time were you able to practice *Wu Ming* Meridian Therapy? Did you track it by recording it in the practice chart? How did you feel? What did you notice? When you notice positive changes, do not think "it's all in my mind." Your body is actually responding to an energy shift in Qi. Reinforce your good efforts by reminding yourself that you are beginning to heal the underlying root cause of your weight problem. I hope that makes you feel very positive, even relieved, and happy.

- Don't go cold turkey!! Gradually eliminate certain foods and incorporate others, as recommended in this chapter. Don't berate yourself if you indulge a little bit more than you should, or hang onto some foods more than you should. Acknowledge and encourage yourself for the good things you've done and move on.

- Notice the foods that you are letting go of. Which have you decided to stop first?

- Notice what you choose as your favorite food and how it tastes. Take great pleasure in this. Do not feel guilty. In fact, try to give up feeling guilty at all about food. Are you one of those dieters who has a constant running monologue about food in your head? You can take comfort in knowing that The Dragon's Way has helped many participants eliminate that awful, mental merry-go-round of constantly bargaining over what foods you will and won't, can and can't eat.

- As you gain more knowledge and become better educated about your body and how it works from the TCM perspective, you should understand why it may well have been impossible for you to lose weight for good with any diet program you've tried before. Remember, you may not want to eat the same foods you love today again; so be prepared to enjoy what you have in front of you.

- Are you someone who's relied on drinking water throughout the day and night? This is something that you'll also gradually give up. How do you feel as you stop drinking so much water?
- Switch to warm foods and drink. Notice how your stomach feels when you drink something cool or warm.
- Take a good look at the emotion(s) that ruled this week. Are you more angry? Sad? Happy? Or have you run a gamut of emotions? Are your spirits high or low or somewhere in between? Did you find those special times and places where you can take a few minutes out for yourself to heal and become peaceful? Note these in your TCM Self-Healing Journal. Incidentally, when you take these special healing breaks for yourself, all you have to do is sit quietly with your eyes closed and breathe normally for just a few minutes.
- A tree or flower reaches its highest peak of Qi or energy when its buds begin to open. Buy yourself a bouquet of flowers this week and try to connect with this beautiful gift of nature. Even one flower can help you reconnect with nature's real Qi. Do this with love and appreciation, both for yourself and for your own role in nature.

THE DRAGON'S WAY CHECKLIST I

Your responses to the following questions will assist you in keeping track of your healing progress in The Dragon's Way program. At the end of six weeks, you will fill out another checklist, so that you can more easily assess the gains you've made over the course of this effort.

Here's one participant's perspective on the many symptoms listed below.

Twenty-six years of teaching can take its toll, especially in accumulated stress-related symptoms. I didn't realize how my lack of energy was gradually causing stress to destroy my health. This program taught me how to take care of myself in a new way. A friend of mine urged me to take this program. I came to it knowing nothing about TCM. What really got my attention was the first TCM checklist I filled out. Looking at it, I realized that I had listed more than twenty different symptoms that were bothering me almost daily: fatigue, depression, nervousness, worry, back pain, dizziness, loss of sexual interest, and muscle tension, and more. What an eye opener! Gradually, I had lost my good health without even realizing it. I was determined to get it back . . . and I did. First I started eating for my stomach, not my mouth. Then I practiced Qigong every day. I took off fifteen pounds, which was great. Then I was able to check off significant improvement in seventeen of the twenty problems that were affecting my health: digestive problems, bloat, nervousness, back pain, muscle tension, dry mouth, cold hands and feet, dizziness, fatigue and depression, and more. This really convinced me of how special this program is.

ANNA J., 48-YEAR-OLD HIGH SCHOOL TEACHER

THE DRAGON'S WAY CHECKLIST I

Symptom	No symptom	Mild	Moderate	Severe
Fatigue	____	____	____	____
Dizziness	____	____	____	____
Palpitations	____	____	____	____
Night sweats	____	____	____	____
Shortness of breath	____	____	____	____
Chest pain	____	____	____	____
Back pain	____	____	____	____
Muscle tension	____	____	____	____
Loss of appetite	____	____	____	____
Abdominal distension	____	____	____	____
Headache	____	____	____	____
Stomachache	____	____	____	____
Diarrhea	____	____	____	____
Constipation	____	____	____	____
Skin rash	____	____	____	____
Dry mouth	____	____	____	____
Insomnia	____	____	____	____
Racing heart	____	____	____	____
Bone pain	____	____	____	____
Joint pain	____	____	____	____
Upset stomach or nausea	____	____	____	____
Sweaty hands	____	____	____	____
Difficulty sleeping	____	____	____	____

Symptom	No symptom	Mild	Moderate	Severe
Irritability or restlessness	____	____	____	____
Depression	____	____	____	____
Nightmares	____	____	____	____
Nervousness	____	____	____	____
Angry moods	____	____	____	____
Worrying	____	____	____	____
Loss of sexual interest	____	____	____	____
Forgetting information	____	____	____	____
Frequent urination	____	____	____	____
Cold hands and feet	____	____	____	____
Heartburn	____	____	____	____
Vaginal discharge	____	____	____	____
Irregular menses	____	____	____	____
Hot flashes	____	____	____	____

CHAPTER 6

WEEK 2:
Breaking Down the Internal "Garbage" and Building Up Your Qi

Now is the time to begin cleaning out the accumulated internal "garbage" as I call it and building up your Qi. This is not a physical detox effort, but takes place at the energy level. We will clear out and cleanse stagnating Qi. This is something that you will do each day with The Dragon's Way Qigong movements. Beginning with this week, I recommend you eat the healing foods and meals suggested.

This week you should continue to follow the recommendations for changing your eating habits. Avoid drinking cold fluids; avoid eating raw vegetables; eat only cooked vegetables (any form of cooking except deep frying and barbecuing will do), and roasted or toasted walnuts or pine nuts. Given the complexity of the digestive process, try to eat dinner before 7:00 or 8:00 P.M. Eat the heaviest foods only in the morning or early afternoon. If you are used to drinking a lot of water, please stop! Once again, you will learn that TCM has a very different view of certain practices that Westerners believe are healthy. You may be surprised at this information. Drink room-temperature water (never cold water) only when you are thirsty.

Learn the remaining five *Wu Ming* Meridian Therapy Qigong movements, and start practicing all ten movements daily.

The TCM lesson for this week will cover The Five Element Theory, the ancient Chinese view of life's web. We'll also begin a discussion about each of your five major organs. This week you'll learn a lot about your liver and the way it is supposed to function, what harms it as well as what heals it. Most important, you'll learn how your lifestyle can affect the healthy function of this vital organ and cause your body to pile on the extra pounds.

During this week, continue with The Dragon's Way Recommended Eating for Healing Plan. If you want The Dragon's Way to work for you, find as many opportunities as you can to practice *Wu Ming* Meridian Therapy Qigong. It is essential for you to understand that what makes The Dragon's Way work is the Qigong. *The foods (and any of our herbs you may have included in your program) are secondary.*

You're about to begin Week 2. How do you feel so far? By now you should have a week's worth of experience with the *Wu Ming* Meridian Therapy Qigong movements. You should also have gradually changed what you have been eating and drinking.

I never like to tell people how they are going to react to this new energy practice and consuming healing foods, but perhaps you have started to feel some changes already. TCM believes every person is unique; so each of us acts and reacts differently to any given set of circumstances. Although you may not see it yet, if you are doing these things, I believe that you have begun to break down what I call your internal "garbage."

Some participants report that they feel a big burst of energy after the first week; many do not feel anything. Some feel a little testy; others say they are exhilarated. There is no right or wrong response. This journey is all about you, your body and its own very particular needs. So pay close attention to how *you* feel and any messages that your body (not your mind!) is sending you as you heal.

When I began Week 2, I found it pretty easy. I have been a vegetarian for about ten years now, so the transition to The Dragon's Way wasn't too hard. I decided to eliminate most carbohydrates and I must admit that I did miss my pasta!

SUSAN L., 32-YEAR-OLD HEALTH FOOD STORE EMPLOYEE

Early on, I found eating just the recommended foods to be a little difficult. The thing is, I'm not a very good cook, and I just didn't have a clue about where to begin. When I got the recipes, that helped a lot. I did do the Qigong, however. The exercises and breathing helped me work through any hunger I had. I also decided to eat extra portions when I needed to satisfy my appetite. Dr. Lu said that we shouldn't be unhappy and deprive ourselves. I guess it didn't matter because I lost twelve pounds and at least seven inches overall anyway.

BILL S., 47-YEAR-OLD FILM PRODUCER

PRACTICING THE SELF-HEALING QIGONG MOVEMENTS

By now, you and your body have gotten to know the first five movements of *Wu Ming* Meridian Therapy. Each meridian stretch has been designed to help your organs function in harmony and increase and strengthen your overall Qi. Each movement targets a particular meridian, also known as an energy channel or pathway, that is connected to a specific organ so that you can unblock stagnating Qi and restore its free flow. (Like the invisible shipping lanes at sea or highways in the sky over which airplanes travel, these pathways in your body bring Qi and its messages to all its structures to provide power to support the functions that keep you alive and well.)

Most Western people recognize the term "meridian" in connection with acupuncture. TCM uses acupuncture to disperse blocked Qi in the meridian passageways by inserting needles at key points along these energy routes. As your Qigong practice develops, you will gradually help release your own Qi (everyone has Qi; without it, you wouldn't be alive) and begin to experience many health benefits from these ancient self-healing movements.

During Week 2, learn the five remaining Dragon's Way movements and add them into your practice. Taken together, these ten ancient movements create a self-healing practice session of about twenty minutes. The more you practice, the more you'll gain.

Number 5: The Dragon Looks at His Tail
Number 6: The Dragon Taps His Foot
Number 7: Rocking the Baby Dragon
Number 8: The Dragon Kicks Backward
Number 9: The Dragon Rises From the Ocean

Descriptions of and instructions for these Qigong movements are found in Chapter 3. Remember, maximum benefit can be gained from practicing in the morning and at night. However, the *quality* of your practice is much more important than quantity. So if you have a single, quality practice of fifteen to twenty minutes, that's much more productive than feeling that you have to do these movements a second time that same day. The most important thing is to do them—even if it's only two of them for five minutes apiece. But I urge you to do your best to commit to a routine where you can practice the full set of ten movements daily. In addition, be smart; look for every opportunity to do one or more of these movements. Do them while you're waiting for a bus, or when you're watching television. You can even do them while you're talking on the phone; just get up and do *The Dragon Kicks Forward* (#2) or *Backward* (#8).

The Qigong is the best thing about The Dragon's Way. The good news is that it will change your life. The bad news? It will change your life. Why is this bad news? Because the program is so powerful that it literally wakes you up to the reality of your own life and lifestyle. You begin to challenge some of your lifelong habits. What was once comfortable may become uncomfortable. Change is difficult, but I am grateful to The Dragon's Way. It really did change my life.

ROBERT S., 46-YEAR-OLD INSURANCE BROKER

TAKING THE PLUNGE: EATING FOR HEALING

By the start of Week 2, you should have eliminated meat, dairy products, raw vegetables and salads, bread, and other high carbohydrates from your diet. When I run The Dragon's Way, I usually ask participants to give up pasta or rice for the six-week period, but I've allowed a half-cup of either on the plan in this book. Have you avoided drinking cold fluids? Soy products? Have you stopped drinking water frequently? Remember, I'd like you to put away those water bottles and only drink when you *feel* you are thirsty. Listen to your body and not your mind.

If so, you are ready to take the plunge.

As you can see from the chart of Recommended Healing Foods, there is a variety of fruits and vegetables to choose from. I always tell Dragon's Way participants to select good quality foods. Don't rush yourself when you go to the grocery store, and don't pick up the first red apple you see. Test yourself. Try to become calm and peaceful. Trust your own instincts. I tell all my Dragon's Way participants: "Please, listen to your body." If you're beginning to tune into your intuition, your hand will naturally go to the fruit or vegetable your body wants. Try it; see for yourself, You might be very surprised at how smart your own body is. Listen to that built-in intelligence radar you were born with.

You might find the following very interesting. This is a basic theory of TCM knowledge that has been successfully applied to health problems for millennia. Today it is especially relevant to issues of weight management. According to TCM, here's what happens when you ingest anything. First food enters your stomach, where the spleen helps to "ripe and rotten" it, as the ancient medical text, the *Nei Jing*, says. This mixture becomes a nutritive essence called *"gu"* Qi. This *"gu"* Qi then gets sent up to your lung (yes, your lung!), which helps distribute the essence to the specific organs that should receive it. Most likely you've never learned about the lung's role in processing food. I think you can immediately grasp why smoking has certain effects on weight.

Let's see what happens when you stir-fry a delicious meal of eggplant, green peppers, plum tomatoes, ginger, garlic, and scallions with sesame oil. Certainly, you do gain all the physical properties of these foods, but you've also received something beyond this. You've received the intangible, (unmeasurable for scientific instruments thus far) yet real power of the Qi of each of these foods. Similar to a little subway car or a small missile, the Qi of each food zips along one of the meridians to enter the organ with which it has a healing relationship.

There it helps support the organ that matches with its healing vibration. The essence of the eggplant, green peppers, and scallions goes directly to your liver. The essence of the plum tomatoes goes to your heart. Ginger and garlic essence goes to your stomach; the essence of the sesame oil goes to your kidney. This one delicious dish can help four of your organs gain a healing benefit.

As you can see, eating for healing is a way for you to use food for its natural purpose, as a source of Qi. This additional Qi can then accrue to the Qi you are building with the Qi-gong, as well as the Qi you are saving by reducing or eliminating stress. And all this extra Qi can be applied to rebalancing your organs and getting them back into a harmonious relationship with each other. Now you're finally healing the root cause of your excess weight. Try to let your anxieties and misunderstandings about food and its role in your life ease away. Eating for healing is a way to learn about yourself as an integrated whole. By the end of these six weeks of your Dragon's Way adventure, you'll have a very good sense about the unique value each food has for balancing your body and its organs. You'll also know how to relate to yourself as a complete holistic energy system consisting of body, mind, spirit, and emotions—with all the parts in constant communication with the other parts. We should never underestimate the wonderful miracle that we are!

TCM'S TOP FIVE FAVORITE FOODS FOR ELIMINATING EXCESS WEIGHT

When we think about fresh food as healing Qi, we see that there is a wide selection to choose from. This week, we will focus on five very useful foods that can help you discard excess weight. The first is eggplant.

Eggplant

Eggplant has the power to balance internal Qi. It is particularly good for harmonizing the Qi of your liver so that it can work more efficiently with its sister organs. Eggplant also has the ability to lower cholesterol. So be sure to eat more than just one small slice! Don't worry about which kind of eggplant to select. There are many different ones, and they're all good for you. If you can ever find white eggplants (readily available in the fall), their Qi is especially good for weight loss purposes, even though they are often more expensive.

Bamboo Shoots

Bamboo shoots are a great healing food. They are especially good for helping the stomach work more smoothly and improving the digestive function. Most likely, you will find bamboo shoots that are canned. They are usually available in most supermarkets in the Chinese food section.

Mushrooms

Next on the list are mushrooms, especially fresh ones. There are many different types of mushrooms and their flavors vary from mild to quite "earthy." The essence of mushrooms goes to both the lung and the stomach. These edible fungi are food that can help prevent cancer. They are all good for you and easily lend themselves to almost any style of cooking. They are fun to experiment with. The only rule I have about mushrooms is that they must be cooked. I strongly recommend that you avoid eating raw mushrooms. Mushrooms are a fungus and carry a different kind of Qi. If your digestive system is not too strong, eating this food raw can cause problems, such as food poisoning.

Eggplant, bamboo shoots, and mushrooms are especially helpful for supporting all your organ systems as you shed excess weight. Try making them a regular part of the meals you prepare during the six-week program and even after you're finished.

Watermelon

The next healing food on the TCM top five favorites list is watermelon. TCM practitioners have prescribed this fruit as part of a medicated diet over the course of many centuries, and still do today. I consider it the most important food you will eat during this entire program. Have watermelon juice as often as possible during The Dragon's Way, because it has a tremendous healing and medicinal purpose for a person who wants to get rid of excess weight. One of its great powers is that it can relieve internal heat. Watermelon is also a good diuretic and is excellent for strengthening the function of your stomach and spleen.

If you juice watermelon, be sure to include some of the white and green parts of the rind as well as the seeds. If you don't have a juicer, you can cut up pieces into small chunks and put them in a blender. Check to see that your blender is strong enough to break down the seeds; otherwise, eliminate this part. If you can, drink watermelon juice every day. For a change of pace, try the yellow watermelon that is becoming more readily available. Cantaloupe and other melons do not have the same healing ability and Qi as watermelon. Because they cannot give you the same benefit, I recommend that you do not substitute them for watermelon juice. If you'd like to try different ways of eating watermelon, experiment with cooking it—sautéing or frying this fruit produces interesting tastes and dishes. Try our special delicious sweet and sour watermelon in The Dragon's Feast in Chapter 12.

Bee Pollen

Another food that's particularly beneficial for balancing your body is bee pollen. You might try several varieties and keep a record of which ones you like the most. I prefer the granular, raw bee pollen. You can find it in the refrigerated section of many health food stores. At first, start with a half teaspoon of bee pollen mixed in juice and gradually increase the amount until you are consuming at least two teaspoons a day. Less than that usually does not have any healing effect. From an energy viewpoint, when you eat bee pollen, you take in the healthy essence that the bees gather from fresh flowers. Bees always go to fresh, healthy flowers, not to weak or dying ones. Bee pollen is also beneficial for strengthening the function of the heart, kidney, and stomach.

TCM LESSON OF THE WEEK: THE FIVE ELEMENT THEORY AND LEARNING ABOUT THE LIVER

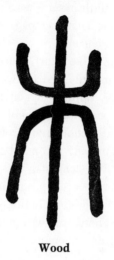

Wood

The Five Element Theory: Ancient World View of Life's Web

The Five Element Theory is one of the oldest theories of how the Universe operates. Ancient TCM doctors learned how to apply its principles in their medical practice. Although The Five Element Theory is described in many TCM medical textbooks, most Westerners are not aware that it is also an intrinsic aspect of Chinese culture, where it forms the foundation of healing disciplines like Feng Shui pronounced (*fung schway*), the art of the place and placement of things, the I Ching pronounced (*eee ching*), and the martial arts. This powerful theory of connections was passed to ancient people who had a very different relationship with and sensitivity to nature than we do today. They were able to tune into things on a deep energetic level that is almost impossible to achieve in our overstimulated world.

They also had a profound understanding that nothing in the Universe lives a separate life. Everything is connected.

The Five Element Theory says that everything is related to some other thing and all things are woven together into a seamless whole. Look at the chart on page 133 so you can better appreciate this ancient wisdom.

As you can see from the chart, there are five circles. Each of the five circles represents one of five elements: wood, fire, earth, metal, and water. Within each circle are other things that correspond with that particular element: a season, a climate or environmental factor, direction, and a color. According to TCM, all aspects of the human body and mind are also related by their nature to one of the five elements. This includes not only the principal organs—liver, heart, spleen, lung, and kidney—but every other part of the body, including emotions, and the five aspects of the soul. Therefore, within each circle is also an organ, its partner organ, an emotion, a taste, a sound, and a sense organ.

Take time to study The Five Element Theory Chart now. Refer to it as often as possible. The longer you study it, the more fascinating the discoveries you might make. Do you see a season in which you always seem to get sick? Do you see an "opening" or tissue that always causes you health problems? Most of all, for people carrying excess weight, do you see an emotion that particularly affects you? What organ is it connected to? If you answered "anger" and "the liver," or "overthinking or worry" and the "spleen," you are not alone.

To understand how a TCM practitioner uses The Five Element Theory in diagnosis and treatment, the first thing you must understand is that although each of the five elements has its own individual system, all of them have an inseparable connection to each other. These connections are indicated by the solid and broken lines linking each of the circles and therefore each of the organs. For the whole system to function in har-

CLASSIFICATION OF THINGS ACCORDING TO THE THEORY OF THE FIVE ELEMENTS

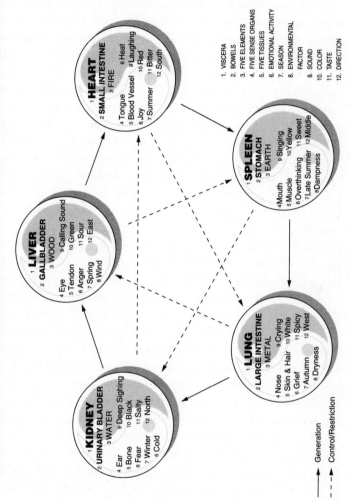

mony, two dynamic relationships must operate smoothly. TCM calls these relationships *generation* and *control.*

It is important to understand that the Five Elements themselves are also not inert substances. They are fundamental energies in nature, and they too, like yin and yang, are continually in motion. Each element generates—or gives birth to—another. That's what we mean by *generation.* In TCM, these element pairs are known as mother and child. This relationship operates just like a real mother and child. For example, unless the mother puts certain limits on her child, she or he would be out of control! I think you can begin to see and appreciate what this means. I also want to emphasize that this is not an abstract concept. This is the way your body operates in reality. When I tell my patients these things, so many of them exclaim, "I never heard that." Or, "I wish I had understood these things a long time ago."

Each element also restrains or *controls* another. The right amount of control keeps all the elements in proper proportion and balance. Without the function of control, generation would be excessive or too much. This kind of interaction enables all the elements—and all the other aspects of the organ listed in each circle, including the organs—to work as one harmonious system. From the health perspective, if these relationships are balanced, you feel well and strong; if any of the relationships become unbalanced, you will suffer from various discomforts and health problems. This is true even if these conditions are not indicated on your scientific tests or do not appear on scientific imaging devices! If you have this experience, you are not imagining that you are not well. You are hearing and feeling that your body is out of balance. TCM practitioners are trained to recognize and address imbalances in a person's Qi and the resulting symptoms.

Let's follow the elemental circles together so you can understand them a little better. Start with the circle that contains the element water. TCM identifies water as the mother (or the generator because it takes water to nourish the trees) of wood (likewise wood is the child of water). Now, follow the dotted arrow from the water circle. You can see that water also has another job or function. It controls the element of fire (that makes sense, because water puts out fire). If we start at the circle that contains the element wood, you can see that it is the mother of fire. Following the dotted arrow across, you can see that wood controls the earth, and so on. Each of the other categories of things inside these five circles has the same relationships of generation and control as the elements themselves do. Study the organs within each circle and begin to learn which ones generate which organs and which ones control which organ. The more you study this complex system, the more insight you will gain into how your body really functions.

Now we can take The Five Element Theory one step further as we look at the whole human body. As I said before, all aspects of the human body and mind are also related by their nature to one of the five elements. So if we again look at the circle with the element of water, we find the kidney there. Following the same pattern as above, you can see that the kidney is the mother of the liver (the liver, then, is the child of the kidney). This is nature's pattern of generation between these two organs. If we follow the dotted arrow from the circle with the element of water, you can see that the Qi of the kidney controls the Qi of the heart.

Following this ancient blueprint, here's what we find:

MOTHER AND CHILD RELATIONSHIPS

- The kidney is the mother of the liver.
- The liver is the mother of the heart.
- The heart is the mother of the spleen.
- The spleen is the mother of the lung.
- The lung is the mother of the kidney.

CONTROL RELATIONSHIPS

- The kidney controls the heart.
- The heart controls the lung.
- The lung controls the liver.
- The liver controls the spleen.
- The spleen controls the kidney.

Now that you understand who are the mother organs and who are the children organs and which organs control the other, you're probably wondering how this framework applies to health and weight gain. Let's begin by looking at the organ most responsible for excess weight—the liver.

THE LIVER AND THE FIVE ELEMENT THEORY

According to TCM, the liver's job is to keep the flow of your body's Qi and blood, as well as your emotions, running smoothly. Yet all too often, the villain of modern life—stress—causes Qi to stop flowing freely and to get stuck, or stagnate, in your body, where it prevents the liver from functioning properly. Similar to a game of dominos, a poorly functioning liver can then have a profound negative effect on your other organs.

Look again at The Five Element Theory Chart. You see that the liver *controls* the spleen. Therefore, in order to have good digestion, the liver must exert the proper amount of control on the stomach. Too much or too little control causes problems. You may suffer from abdominal distension or indigestion; you may burp a lot and have a sour taste in your mouth (the taste associated with the liver). Or you may gain weight.

Therefore, what presents itself or appears as a stomach problem is really being generated by a liver function disorder. Simply put, the liver isn't functioning or working the way it should and a problem then arises somewhere else, like the stomach or spleen. Following is one woman's struggle with a liver dysfunction.

> *I was desperate before I started this program. My digestion was pretty poor. It made me feel heavy, bloated, and sluggish all day long. I had a stubborn skin rash. Most disturbing for me were the recurring nightmares and the nervousness that I just couldn't shake. What I found was a great program and a great learning experience. Best of all, I could put the information into practice right away. I practiced the* Wu Ming *Meridian Therapy Qigong every day. And I must say, for me, they really are "therapy"! I actually enjoy eating foods from the energy healing list. The overall effect of the program on my health has been incredible. Now, I feel much clearer and lighter. I'm energized and sleep well. My digestion is so much better and the bloated feeling is gone. The skin rash disappeared around the fifth week, and I'm relieved to say that the nightmares and nervousness have gone away. I "gave up" thirteen pounds in six weeks without thinking about my weight. I received so much benefit from this program. These Qigong movements and these new ways of viewing health are a permanent part of my life.*
>
> LESLIE B., 40-YEAR-OLD DEPARTMENT MANAGER

So let's take a closer look at the liver circle and see what TCM has to say about this organ.

- The gallbladder is the partner organ of the liver.
- Wood is the liver's corresponding element because, like a long slender wooden bamboo stalk, the liver's Qi likes to move upward and outward freely. The roots are nourished by the earth, which is in the circle of the spleen.
- The eye is the sense organ related to the liver. So if you have eye problems, it may be a sign that deep down your liver is not functioning smoothly.

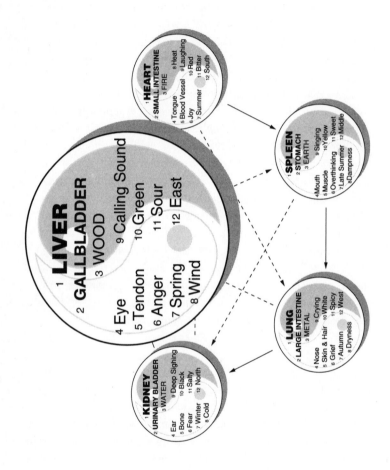

- The tendons are the "tissue" or "sinew" associated with the liver. TCM says strength comes from tendons, not muscles. If you want to be truly strong for your whole life, take a page from the cat's book. It has strength, agility and flexibility, but it does not have a huge muscle mass. A cow is an animal with giant muscle mass, but little real strength. Do you want to be like a cat or a cow?
- Anger is the emotion associated with the liver. Therefore, if you often feel irritable, have trouble unwinding from the day's activities, are easy to anger, have trouble "going with the flow," and letting things go, or have difficulty with your ability to reason, you are experiencing a liver function problem. Likewise, these negative emotions, especially if chronic or excessive, can seriously unbalance the function of your liver.
- Wind is the environmental factor associated with the liver.
- Spring is the season of the liver.
- East is its direction (so face east when you are doing the Qigong movements if you have liver problems).
- Green is the color connected to the liver (so wear green in the liver's season, spring!).
- Sour is the taste associated with the liver. If you have a sour taste in your mouth all the time or crave sour food, your liver is talking to you and asking you to rebalance its function.

There are so many things you can learn from The Five Element Theory. Take a look again at the liver circle. You'll see that the season related to this organ is spring. Spring is an exciting time for most people. It's when nature awakens from winter's rest and a sense of renewal fills the air. You and everything else are bursting with energy! Yet quite often, people get allergies, high blood pressure is aggravated, or other ailments appear with the arrival of spring. Why? Because when a season's energy or Qi changes, your body must also match with these cycles of Universal change. If you can't, you will become sick. When the seasons change, you are at your most vulnerable. Therefore, if your life is always very stressful it has an affect on the amount of Qi you have available to deal with these changes, and health problems will appear in the season of the liver, which is spring. Though your liver would like to pursue its natural course of "going with the flow," unfortunately, it just can't. Its Qi gets "stuck" and needs to be freed.

So in spite of the good feelings that this season fosters, I always tell people to stay calm during the spring. Take things easy. Go slow. Take a nice long walk in the park or do other gentle exercises. Don't get too caught up in spring's intense new energies.

Also, don't be fooled by the burst of change. Often the weather fluctuates in the spring so that it is cool one day, then hot, then cool again. To keep up with these weather changes, we have a tendency to wear less clothing or dress in layers, removing jackets and sweaters because it feels warm. While this seems like the logical thing to do, I always tell my patients that it's not such a good idea. Why? Because the true essence of spring is cold, and even if the temperature rises, you must use up your Qi to stay warm. Remember, TCM is a holistic medical system whose foundation is Qi. According to TCM, everything is about Qi or energy and how we use it. Therefore, I urge you to be smart and not to deplete your Qi to stay warm, especially if you are trying to eliminate excess weight. It's much simpler and more energy-efficient to wear an extra sweater or jacket until the cold essence of spring changes to the warmth of summer. Now that you know about saving and using your Qi for healing purposes, it makes so much more sense to cooperate with nature, rather than challenge it, and end up wasting the very Qi you have worked so hard to acquire.

Getting back to the liver, many people want to know how they can tell if their liver is working well. Here are some common signs that would tell me as a TCM practitioner that you have problems with your liver function. I would like to be very clear that we are not talking about your physical organ, we are referring to the way your liver performs the tasks that are ingrained or programmed in the organ itself. If you've had your liver tested and you've been told that it is perfect, that's very good; however, if you exhibit any of the following signs, then you should understand that your liver is not functioning properly. A well-trained TCM practitioner immediately recognizes these signs of liver dysfunction:

1. Brittle fingernails that break easily and have little or no half moons.
2. Blurred vision; eyes that are dry, red and/or swollen, burn, or tear easily. TCM considers tears to be the fluid of the liver; these eye problems arise when this organ's function is disturbed.
3. Tendon problems. It also works the other way around; problems with the tendons affect the liver's ability to function properly—which is why I tell patients and students alike to stay away from fast and hard exercises that overwork or overstretch the tendons, causing them eventually to lose their flexibility.
4. Migraine headaches (especially on either side).
5. Indigestion and bloating.
6. Excess weight.
7. Angry moods.
8. Constantly being stressed out.
9. Yeast infections.
10. *Any* menstrual/PMS/menopausal problems.
11. Cold hands and feet. Remember, it's the liver's responsibility to keep your blood flowing smoothly, and if it's not doing its job, your circulation is compromised.
12. Bruises easily (blood circulation is compromised).
13. Bad breath.
14. Shaking disorders such as Parkinson's disease.

15. Arthritis that moves throughout the body. TCM says that this condition can be caused by overexposure to the wind. An example of how this happens is by wearing short skirts in the winter or in cold windy weather, allowing the wind to enter the meridians of the legs.

Knowing what you do now about strengthening the liver and its Qi, here are some foods that will help this vital organ function more smoothly and support you in the healing process:

Bamboo shoots
Bee pollen
Broccoli rabe
Dandelion greens
Eggplant
Fennel
Garlic
Ginger
Lemon
Lotus
Safflower oil
Scallions
Vinegar

MY MESSAGE FOR YOU FOR WEEK 2

This coming week might still feel a little difficult while you adjust to the change in foods and find a way to integrate Qigong movements into your daily routine. You are also absorbing a lot of new ideas about how your body works and about TCM. Once you've gotten through the week, you should be fine. Try to go through this week "on the program." Eat meals when you should; drink water only when you're thirsty; get enough sleep; practice Qigong daily; stay peaceful and calm. Be happy that you are really addressing the root cause of your weight issues. Remember, this is a time to persevere and enjoy the challenge. Your health and your body are in good hands—your own.

Every one of you reading this book can use these new tools to let go of excess weight and enhance the quality of your life. You each have the one quality that you most need to do this: belief in your own healing abilities. Even if you read that sentence and you have some doubts, your intuition has led you to this knowledge. You've come this far in life and are seeking new solutions for the excess baggage you are carrying. You are willing to look at different possibilities. This takes trust, curiosity and dedication.

Have a peaceful week. Take good care of yourself.

WEEK 2: HELPFUL HINTS FOR GETTING THROUGH THIS WEEK

- If you start to feel hungry, practice *The Dragon Rises From the Ocean* (#9) and/or *The Dragon Stands Between Heaven and Earth* (#10). If that doesn't help enough, practice the Reverse Breathing Meditation in Chapter 2.
- Practice the *Wu Ming* Meridian Therapy movements every day, and try to incorporate them into your daily life. For example, do *The Dragon Twists (#3)* while you're at the copy machine, or waiting for a bus, or on a line at the supermarket. Practice *The Dragon Kicks Backward* (#2) or *Forward* (#8) while you're watching TV. Or take a five-minute break from your computer and *Rock the Baby Dragon* (#7).
- Start identifying stressful situations and eliminate them from your life. If that's not possible, here are my favorite time-tested TCM ways of relieving stress:

  ◊ Break glass bottles (preferably green, the liver's color vibration) in a safe place, smash raw eggs, or stomp on raw potatoes (with your shoes on) or slowly push your toe into a fully inflated balloon until it bursts and you have the feeling that something has been relieved!

◊ Get a hairbrush with plastic bristles. With the bristle side down, hit the insides of your legs in a downward motion only—at least two minutes on each leg. This helps stimulates the liver meridians that run through this area.

◊ Scream at the top of your lungs (works very well in your car!).

◊ Stop drinking alcohol; it can put a lot of stress on the liver.

◊ Learn how to let things go.

• Try these two simple breathing exercises and energy techniques to deal with stress. They can also help control hunger:

◊ Close your eyes and picture yourself walking in a flower garden. Look around the garden and see your favorite flower in a beautiful shade of bright, rich yellow. The garden is now filled only with your favorite flower in this beautiful yellow color. You look around the garden and notice that of all the flowers you choose one that, at this very moment, is at its peak point of beauty. It is staying right there at that point. This is the point of its highest power, when the flower has the most Qi. It is at its peak moment. That's where you want to be at this very moment also—open, in touch with your strongest Qi. Breathe in all the Universal energy in this flower. Breathe it in quietly for five to ten minutes.

◊ Sit with your back straight and not touching the back of the chair. TCM believes that female and male energy cycles run in seven- and eight-year periods, respectively. If you are female, close your eyes and picture yourself before you were seven years old; if you are a male, before you were eight years old. Breathe in and out slowly and deeply without straining. Remember what you looked like at this young age as you calmly breathe in and out. See your face. Notice how clear your face is. See your eyes. Notice how bright they are at this time. Notice your healthy, shiny hair. See your whole body. Remember how supple it felt. Keep breathing in and out slowly and deeply. Let go of this picture. Keep your eyes closed and breathe slowly in and out. Keep your back straight and stay relaxed. Now picture yourself at the happiest time in your life, at any age. Continue breathing slowly and calmly in and out. Everyone has had a happy time. It doesn't matter which one you choose. Remember how you looked. Remember how you felt. Let yourself feel this good feeling again. Breathe deeply and calmly in and out as you experience this happy feeling. There is no need to hurry. You are sitting straight. Breathe in deeply and let this good feeling fill your whole body. Breathe in and relax even more as you breathe out. Breathe this happy feeling in and relax even more as you breathe out. Breathe in and out naturally. Now see yourself walking in a flower garden. You see your favorite flower in front of you. You can smell the flower and you can feel its Qi. Breathe the aroma of your favorite flower in deeply and breathe out gently. Make a wish. Make a big wish. For women, breathe in and out seven times; for men, eight times. Slowly open your eyes.

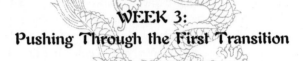

CHAPTER 7
WEEK 3:
Pushing Through the First Transition

*W*EEK 3 is almost always a pivotal week for The Dragon's Way. This is when a number of things can start to change—your emotions, your eating habits and your desires, and for many people, the body itself. Some people have difficulty during the third and fourth weeks. Why? If you've been practicing the *Wu Ming* Meridian Therapy Qigong daily, this is the time of energy transition. Congratulate yourself. Your body is literally beginning to "wake up." It's very important to conserve your awakening Qi for healing your excess weight condition at this time. Don't go out and join a gym or think that you can go marathon mall shopping on the weekend. Be kind to yourself and rest as much as you possibly can during The Dragon's Way. My patients and our participants always struggle with this concept because there is very little in our Western lifestyles that encourages us to remain calm, and to rest and relax. Many people are afraid of being perceived as lazy. Don't buy this cultural conditioning for a second! Try to understand that healing yourself is the most important activity you can do. Then believe it. Remember that what makes The Dragon's Way work is the Qigong. *The foods and herbs are secondary.* In the TCM lesson of the week, we'll take an in-depth look at the kidney and the central role it plays in your capacity for generating and storing Qi. By this week, you've now gotten to know the *Wu Ming* Meridian Therapy movements and have begun to change your eating patterns, as well as the foods you eat. I also hope that you have begun to take notice of how you select the fruits and vegetables from your grocery store, and are becoming aware of the TCM way of thinking about the healing capabilities of food.

For some people, the first few weeks of The Dragon's Way are an easy uphill climb. For others it is not. In fact, some say that Week 3, in particular, is a time when they feel frustrated and think they may not be eating enough or that there is not an ample variety of foods to choose from. At this point in The Dragon's Way, people have also been known to become cranky about doing the Qigong movements every day, and a few enter into some self-doubt about the program. I've even heard some individuals expressing concern that the things they are doing are "too different." Other people find they are easily annoyed at minor things in their life or have a general feeling of dissatisfaction. This is not a bad sign. In fact, it's a sign from your own body that things are beginning to change deep within at the energy level. Not everyone feels this way, but if you do, you are quite normal. All of these negative thoughts and feelings are connected to liver Qi and liver function.

Remember, the main emotions associated with the liver are anger and stress. When anger and stress are not released we feel depressed, irritable, annoyed, frustrated, or just have a feeling of being stuck. However, as I've told you, a normally functioning liver works to promote emotional stability. Just as the liver's function is to keep blood and Qi circulating smoothly, it is also responsible for the even flow of emotions. Because TCM has the comprehensive framework of The Five Element Theory, it can trace unbalanced emotions directly to a particular organ. This emotional aspect is often dismissed, ignored, or misunderstood in Western health care. Or, it is understood as the province of the mind, not the body.

As you now know, from the moment you start The Dragon's Way, you begin to awaken the Qi of your body, mind, spirit, and emotions. Your liver—which has been especially affected by the stresses of today's lifestyle—is the organ most likely to respond to or feel these changes first. And sometimes, as it is with many holistic changes, some people may have to take several steps back before they can move forward. If this happens to you, I hope you will be encouraged by reminding yourself that at long last you are working with a program that can really reach deeply into your body and help you correct the root cause of your weight problem. When you do fix it, you might be surprised at the other areas of your health that also improve. You are a holistic being; one change (good or bad) in one aspect of your being will definitely affect another.

As soon as I started The Dragon's Way, I began to feel different. I felt energized in a way that I had never felt before, and after the first week, I was able to wear my wedding ring—something I hadn't been able to do in years. In the end, while I just discarded (not lost!!) a few pounds, I felt terrific. So after the six weeks, I stopped for two, then went back onto The Dragon's Way, in my own way at home. Mostly I concentrated on practicing the Wu Ming *Meridian Therapy movements. The second time around, even more weight dropped, and more inches. . . . The more I healed, the better I felt.*

BARBARA B., 56-YEAR-OLD MARKETING AND SALES MANAGER

QIGONG PRACTICE

By now, you should have been practicing *Wu Ming* Meridian Therapy every day for two weeks. Some of you have undoubtedly begun to notice some changes. Perhaps you feel more energy or that your energy level is higher even throughout the day. You may not be experiencing as many energy fluctuations as you used to, such as being awake and alert for a while and then feeling very tired a few hours later. If you are doing the Qigong movements, that is why. Remember, they are the most powerful healing tool I can teach you. Of course, all of my students want to understand how these movements work. Let me answer this question by telling you about the meridians.

TCM identifies twelve major meridians or energy channels that run through the body. These twelve are part of an extensive invisible energy network. Each of these major meridians is connected to an organ and viscera.

One way of understanding the function of the meridian system is to think about a subway system and streets of a major city. There are subway lines that travel the length and width of the city. Some of these lines are deep below the city streets, while others are closer to the surface. Regardless of where they are, along all the subway routes are station stops that allow access to the city above and its surface network of streets, which provide even further access to travel about town.

In a similar way, some meridians are deeper in the body than others, and, through a variety of channels, they connect with each other and to the body's physical structures—organs, viscera, tissues, skin, nerves, blood vessels, bones, muscles, ligaments, and tendons. The meridians serve as an energy connection and a communications system. It is through the meridian network that Qi reaches all the parts of your body. It is also through the meridian system that the organs, viscera, nerves, etc., send messages to each other almost instantaneously, describing their condition and current needs. Essentially, the meridian system helps control the various functions of the organs, delivers Qi and messages or information throughout the body, and thereby keeps the whole body in a state of balance or equilibrium. Keeping the meridians open, unblocked and in a healthy condition is imperative for the body's self-regulating actions to occur automatically and for us to enjoy good health. But quite often, the Qi that is supposed to hum through these meridians becomes blocked or clogged. When this happens, Qi can stagnate. Then all kinds of things can happen; your body feels tired, achy, ill, or out of sorts. You may get headaches, or have digestive problems, or find it difficult to get a good night's sleep.

Consider what happens at rush hour when heavy traffic backs up and clogs the streets. Cars and buses become crowded together, and traffic begins to slow down. The time to travel from place to place increases with this transportation slowdown. You could say that areas of the city become sluggish. This is similar to what happens in our bodies when our meridians become "clogged." When Qi cannot travel freely and smoothly through a meridian, the areas that are served by that meridian do not receive the proper amount and quality of Qi and the information they need to function properly. Fortunately for us, it is extremely difficult to damage the meridians beyond repair and they can be rehabilitated through healing foods and herbs, acupuncture and acupressure massage, as well as energy practices such as Qigong.

The ancient *Wu Ming* Meridian Therapy taught in The Dragon's Way enables the smooth, even flow of Qi to resume its healthy journey throughout the meridian system. This is a skill that you can learn and use for the rest of your life. Here is an area where you can take responsibility for your own health and healing. Practicing these Qigong movements is true prevention, but *you* have to do the work. You must practice. You might find that some very interesting things happen as your practice continues.

I haven't used a scale in years. I can tell by how my clothes fit if my weight has changed. But I do have a tape measure and I have shrunk eight inches in the past six weeks. My whole body is tighter and firmer. The program taught me a lot about how to take care of myself. My entire outlook has shifted and I've actually experienced the self-healing nature of my body. It's a very exciting feeling. My job as a dispatcher is pretty stressful, but stress doesn't seem to bother me anymore. I get far fewer headaches and my back pain is gone. I sleep much better, my sense of smell and taste is better, in fact, everything is better! This program is amazing.

MARCY L., 45-YEAR-OLD DISPATCHER

If you are finding Week 3 to be especially challenging, *The Dragon Stands Between Heaven and Earth* (#10) is a good movement to do more of this week. This is a time to persevere through those moments of discomfort during this posture. So when you are standing there and feeling tired, don't drop your arms and take a rest. The secret of increasing Qi is this: it is only during the last few seconds of this practice that you can increase your Qi. When are the last few seconds? It is when you feel tired, when you start to feel a little shaky, when you feel a kind of "burn" in your legs or arms, and your mind wants to quit. That is the very time you shouldn't give up. So don't stop. Test yourself. Even if you can only hold the posture for a few more seconds, push yourself *through* this feeling. You will not always experience this feeling when you practice. It's mostly at the beginning, when Qi is beginning to circulate.

How long can you stay in that position even if it is uncomfortable? It is up to you to decide how much you are going to increase you Qi. But I can assure you that if you want to train your body, mind, and spirit to work together as one magnificent system, *The Dragon Stands Between Heaven and Earth* (#10) is the best one to practice. There are many studies in China that discuss the cardiovascular, neurological, and other physical benefits of Qigong. Often when I introduce these movements, particularly the last one, I tell our participants that many people can run on a treadmill for two hours, or run in the park for miles and miles. Yet they cannot stand in this posture for five minutes. Why? Because their body, mind and spirit are not in harmony, and their real Qi or life force is not very strong. They may have physical endurance, but they don't have true strength. What good is all that physical exercise if you're not enhancing your life force? There are numerous studies in China of individuals who have rid themselves of cancer by only doing standing Qigong meditations like *The Dragon Stands Between Heaven and Earth* (#10) for many hours at a time.

EATING FOR HEALING: A NEW WAY TO THINK ABOUT FOOD

For many of you, eating for healing is probably beginning to make sense, and now is the time you should be experimenting with the various recipes in this book. For others, this way of relating to food is still very new.

I hope that you have not been bothered by the familiar voice inside you which says, "I have been cheating . . ." I want you to know that this conversation is not even possible in The Dragon's Way because this program is not a diet. What if you find yourself occasionally eating foods that are not on the program's recommended foods for healing list? Please don't get frustrated, or feel like a failure. You've made a food selection choice and, believe it or not, in the end, strictly sticking to this food plan is not the most critical part of our program.

The Dragon's Way is designed so that the more fully you participate, the greater the benefit you'll receive. It is meant to be a learning experience. I want you to learn how to prevent health problems, how to manage stress, how to think about eating and exercise and spirituality and more, and to discover how to eat for energy and how to understand and respond to your body's unique energy messages. Ultimately, change will occur. How much change will depend on your state of balance or imbalance at the start of the program, as well as your commitment to practicing the energy movements and eating the recommended foods. The time period will vary for each person. Remember, it is *you* who must encourage yourself with positive messages of change.

The more you think of yourself as changing, the more you will. The people who derive the most benefit are those who really believe that they are challenging their excess weight condition and recalling their own healing abilities. That's why I can say with confidence that most people in The Dragon's Way can give up twelve pounds and eight inches in six weeks. I believe you can be one of them. Because you might be experiencing a higher level of change this week, try and capture some of these physical, emotional, and spiritual shifts in your Healing Journal.

FIVE MORE OF MY FAVORITE TCM HEALING FOODS FOR ELIMINATING EXCESS WEIGHT

Here are brief descriptions of the healing properties of five more foods I've chosen for The Dragon's Way.

Celery

Celery's essence is cool. It is very good for increasing stomach Qi and taking the heat out of the body. Too much internal heat can slow down the flow of Qi or cause it to stagnate. Celery can clean out your body and help you release excess water. Also, it can relieve joint pain and promote sound, calm sleep. I always recommend celery for people with diabetes and high blood pressure.

Ginger

TCM recognizes ginger as one of the most powerful foods for healing. I say that because ginger, whose essence is warm, gets rid of cold conditions in the body. Too much internal cold can also slow down the movement of Qi. Think of what cold does. It causes things to constrict, or congeal. With that in mind, it is useful to know that ginger relieves digestive problems, helps liver Qi flow smoothly, and warms the lung.

Scallions

Scallions carry a warm essence. They too benefit the liver and stomach, relieving the body of internal cold conditions. Scallions can help alleviate headaches, and rid the body of colds, skin rashes, menstrual difficulties, and infections. For colds with a headache, runny nose, and chills, I recommend that my patients drink this tea: take the white parts of five scallions, chopped, and two pieces of sliced fresh ginger. Bring them to a boil in two cups of water. Strain, add brown sugar, and drink. Take a hot shower, then wrap yourself in a blanket. Repeat for a few days, if necessary. This will warm you from head to toe and will help drive the cold energy out of your body.

Pears

Pears, on the other hand, have a cool essence. This wonderful fruit helps relieve heat in the lung. Because pears are a little harder to digest than, let's say, an apple, I always tell people to eat a pear if you are hungry during and after The Dragon's Way. It will keep your digestive system engaged and you'll feel more full.

Here's a good recipe for a healing soup that can increase lung Qi and help alleviate coughs in the fall: put a julienne pear, 4–5 sliced almonds, the peel of 1 tangerine and a little honey in 3 cups of water. Simmer slowly for 15 minutes. When finished, remove the tangerine rind and eat for a few days.

Cauliflower

Cauliflower has a neutral essence. I recommend it in The Dragon's Way because TCM uses it to increase kidney Qi and because it is especially good for constipation.

Remember, foods can have more than one healing property,

and for this program, I am especially interested in those that help your liver function more smoothly, and which increase the Qi of your kidney, lung, and spleen.

TCM LESSON OF THE WEEK: THE KIDNEY AND ITS ROLE IN WEIGHT LOSS AND MAINTAINING A HEALTHY BODY

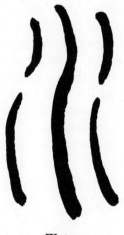

Water

As you learned in Week 2, the ancient Chinese healers saw five sets of interrelated patterns which corresponded to the world around them. These patterns became known as The Five Element Theory.

According to this TCM theory, the role of the kidney is vital. This is the organ where our Inborn Qi—the Qi we inherit at birth—is stored. The kidney holds the key to your energy foundation. It is your whole body's power engine.

As we discussed, we have two kinds of Qi—Inborn and Acquired. They are our savings and checking accounts, respectively. As you can imagine, your energy savings account is strongest when you are born. As you age, the kidney Qi in this account starts to decline. This is simply part of natural law. Everyone's kidney Qi declines over time; that is part of the aging process. For a woman, Qi peaks at fourteen and the energy declines or steps down every seven years until the seventh cycle, when she is forty-nine. At this time, a woman's kidney Qi is almost used up. It's at this time, especially in Western society, that menopausal problems appear. Why? Because kidney Qi is too low to support the other organs.

For a man, Qi peaks at sixteen and then the cycle of decline occurs every eight years until the eighth cycle, or when he is sixty-four. Men then also go through a kind of menopause where various health problems appear. If, at an early age, you can learn how to save Inborn kidney Qi, and maintain a healthy checking account, you can increase the quality and longevity of your life.

Unfortunately, most people don't understand this concept and don't have enough information to live their lives this way. Below is a chart that illustrates how Qi declines over time.

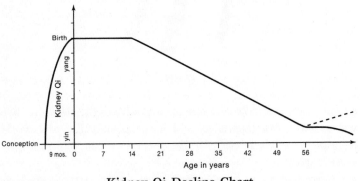

Kidney Qi Decline Chart

Many women in Western culture are affected more than they know by the stress and strain of today's world with its endless pressures and demands and unhealthy lifestyle choices. Their irreplaceable kidney Qi has declined faster than it should for their age because they have used it up. I try very hard to educate my women patients about how to save their Qi before menopause so that they will have fewer problems when they reach this phase of their life. Why? According to TCM, hormone replacement therapy (HRT) or estrogen replacement therapy (ERT) is not necessary because a woman's body has the ability to produce enough hormones for the rest of her life, as long as her kidney and liver function are in balance. If you are interested in more in-depth information on menopause, be sure to read another book in this series, *Traditional Chinese Medicine: A Woman's Guide to a Natural Menopause,* also from Avon Books.

Men, you are not off the hook either. The same is true for you! Everyone has limited Inborn Qi, and unless you've made a concerted effort to conserve it, you too can have problems when you reach the later years of your life.

To learn more about this vital organ, study the kidney's elemental circle on the next page. You can see that:

• The kidney's partner organ is the bladder.

• Its season is winter. So prior to and during the winter months, it's important to eat foods that are especially good for strengthening the kidney.

• The kidney's direction is north (so remember to face north when you're trying to heal your kidney!).

• Water is its element. Accordingly, if the kidney is functioning properly, it performs its normal metabolic function in cooperation with the bladder of ridding the body of excess water. If you are bothered by frequent urination, then you can be sure you have a kidney Qi deficiency.

• The kidney's color is deep blue or black. If you were practicing The Five Element Theory in your life, you would wear these colors to help increase kidney Qi.

• The opening gate to the outside of the body is the ear. Therefore, if you or your child have chronic ear infections, the root cause could be a kidney Qi deficiency. This means that the physical organ may be all right, but the way that it functions, or performs its programmed assignments in the body, is not.

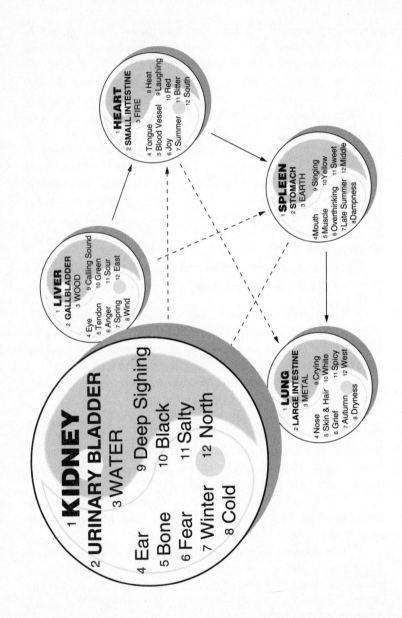

TCM would treat the kidney with herbs to help address these ear infections. If they are chronic, that is a sign that the root cause has not been healed. You should also pay attention if you have tinnitus or ringing in the ears. If there is no physical cause, then it is most likely a kidney Qi deficiency. It is very important to protect your ears, especially during the winter. Be sure to cover them up so that they are not affected by the cold.

• The tissue that the kidney controls is the bone. If your child has delayed tooth growth, or is slow in walking, these are bone-related matters, which means ultimately they are related to the kidney. If you have chronic lower back pain or sore knees, this too is related to deficient kidney Qi. Also, osteoporosis is an indication that kidney Qi is low and not functioning properly. TCM doctors treat all bone problems by addressing the kidney first.

• The emotion associated with the kidney is fear. Panic attacks and nightmares in which you experience great fear are signs of deficient kidney Qi.

• Its environmental factor is cold.

• The taste that goes directly to the kidney is salty. Eating shellfish is very good for your kidney and your bones. I recommend that you eat a lot of shellfish (since you shouldn't eat tablespoons full of salt, you can eat food from the salty sea) if you have a kidney Qi deficiency problem.

Following are some of the most common signs of a kidney that is not functioning properly. TCM would immediately recognize them as problems to pursue for healing:

1. Hair loss
2. Bones that break easily
3. Forgetfulness
4. Frequent urination
5. Thyroid problems
6. High blood pressure
7. Knee pain, heel pain, neck pain, and chronic lower back pain

8. Ringing in the ears
9. Constant thirst
10. Constant cold, especially of the hands and feet
11. Loss of sexual desire
12. Infertility and low sperm count

If you have one or more of the problems listed above, then you know that your kidney Qi already is not functioning properly. If you've tried unsuccessfully to lose weight before The Dragon's Way, you can begin to see why this effort was so difficult. The root cause was not being addressed.

As you've already learned, we are constantly drawing on our savings account of Inborn Qi, and often use its precious funds wastefully. So remember, do everything you can to conserve it. Conservation, if we follow the way of nature, is the most important principle with regard to the kidney. The kidney, as you can see from the above list, corresponds with the season of winter. And think of what happens during the winter. Trees lose their leaves, animals hibernate, birds fly south, and lakes and ponds freeze over. Nature withdraws into herself; she saves her energy and she rests. In the same way, we should follow nature's example. Become more conscious of the value of your Qi foundation and do everything possible to conserve it. This is particularly important if you are trying to lose weight.

Every year, I see many patients who either gain weight or get sick right after the New Year. Why do so many of these people gain weight? It's not necessarily because they've overeaten during the holidays, although they sometimes blame it on that. Interestingly enough, the root cause of their weight gain or illness is the fact that they have mentally, physically, and emotionally overdrawn Qi from their Energy Savings Account.

Eating for healing and strengthening your Acquired Qi can reduce your usage of Inborn Qi.

Here are activities that can waste your special kidney Qi needlessly:

- Exercising too much
- Staying up past midnight
- Drinking cold things on a regular basis
- Taking a cold shower after exercising
- Too much sex

••

TCM HEALING TIP

To remain awake after midnight, your body must spend two to three times the amount of Qi it spends during daytime to keep all the organs functioning. Remember, this is its normal recharge time. So go to sleep before midnight!

••

While it may not be easy to increase kidney Qi, slowing its decline is another matter, and there are many ways you can do this. Here are some of my favorite suggestions.

- Practice the *Wu Ming* Meridian Therapy.
- Be sure you get adequate rest. Sleep helps your body rejuvenate.
- During the winter months, take a vacation to a nice warm place.
- Learn how to sit quietly. Don't always run your body, mind, and spirit at warp speed. I recommend that you listen to restful music or meditate.
- Your ear is the window of your kidney. You can perform self-massage by rubbing your ears until they are nice and warm. This way you can actually stimulate the energy of your whole body.

Following a healthy diet with high-quality, fresh foods is another important step you can take. Below are foods you can eat that can help boost the power of your kidney and rid your body of excess water. It's especially important to make these foods a part of your diet during the winter months, when the kidney is most susceptible to problems. When I lecture, I tell my audiences that Qi is like money in some ways. One way to make money is to earn new money. Another way to make money is to cut expenses. TCM considers it almost impossible to acquire more Inborn Qi, but it is possible to cut our Qi expenditures and conserve our special Qi for longevity.

Here are the healing foods recommended in The Dragon's Way that are especially good for the kidney:

> Bone soup
> Black sesame seed
> Cauliflower
> Cinnamon
> Toasted pine nuts
> Sesame and walnut oils
> Toasted walnuts

Other foods that you should eat to help boost kidney Qi when you've completed the six-week Dragon's Way program are:

> Beans, especially black beans
> Shellfish (shrimp, squid, oysters, lobster, clams)
> Nuts (roast or toast them yourself, or buy commercially dry-roasted products; avoid nuts that are too salty)

MY FINAL THOUGHTS FOR YOU FOR WEEK 3

If you are feeling discouraged in any way during Week 3, remember that this is a common threshold for some participants. If you are feeling terrific, that's normal too. Everyone is different, and every single individual has a unique starting point. If you have not started to lose weight, your body is not ready! But it is in the "processing" mode. Don't be fooled; if you've been practicing *Wu Ming* Meridian Therapy Qigong movements faithfully and you've been eating for healing, as a Qigong master I can tell you that something is happening. It's like when you cook a turkey. How long it takes to finish cooking depends on the size and temperature of the oven. Internally, things are definitely cooking.

So be patient. It's impossible to heal yourself overnight. But even if you don't see changes on the outside, inside things are already changing. Stop and remember all the small, positive changes that you're experiencing. Be sure and note these advances in your Healing Journal. For example, your nightmares may have disappeared. Your insomnia may have improved dramatically. You now may wake up almost every morning feeling refreshed. Your morning headache may have disappeared. Your constipation or bloatedness could be all but eliminated. Your allergies may have stopped giving you as many problems as they did before. Stress doesn't seem to bother you as much. Now, ask yourself, what else has improved? If you're already experiencing these health benefits, but your weight has not changed, don't give up. Your healing needs to go deeper before this symptom starts to disappear. Instead, congratulate yourself. Your healing process has already begun. Try to save Qi whenever and wherever you can. I believe you will see major improvement in the coming week.

•••

WEEK 3: HELPFUL HINTS FOR GETTING THROUGH THE WEEK

- People often want me to tell them how big a portion should be. I never say. You must learn and then decide what is right for you. How will you discover this? Listen to your body and not your mind.
- Eat slowly. All of my Dragon's Way participants get a pair of chopsticks in our program. I suggest using these

chopsticks for every meal. Even these simple Chinese eating utensils reflect the TCM principle of yin and yang—one moves, the other remains stationary. If you don't know how to eat with chopsticks, there is a drawing below that shows you the correct position of the chopsticks and how to hold them. There is also a very important meridian on the moving finger that massages the large intestine while you eat. Someone told me that there is an old Chinese saying: "In ancient times, the Chinese people used to use a fork, but then they became enlightened and began to use chopsticks."

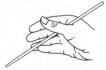

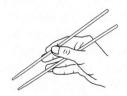

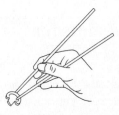

- If you feel frustrated by the foods for healing and feel they are too limiting, remember this program is only for six weeks. Think of it as giving your body a rest. But,

I want to encourage you—do not focus on the food. You have a lifetime to eat whatever you want. And, the good news is that if you do rebalance yourself, you can eat whatever you want after that because your body will tell you what it needs.

- Avoid drinking and eating cold things. Only eat vegetables that are cooked in some way even if you've immersed them in boiling water for a few minutes. Why? Because I want you to save all the healing Qi you can. Even though you may gain slightly more nutrition from raw vegetables, you will save a great deal of Qi by digesting cooked ones.
- Here are some other helpful hints to strengthen kidney Qi:
  ◊ Crawl like a baby! This simple exercise can promote great health benefits such as the relief of joint problems, especially in the knees.
  ◊ Bite your teeth together lightly, fifty times. In TCM, teeth are the "excess" of the bones. Stimulating your teeth can help stimulate your kidney. Do this daily.
  ◊ Rub your ears. Cover each one entirely with your hand and rub them briskly until they feel warm.

• •

Here is another relaxing healing meditation that you can use. You might want to record the following in your own words and play them back while you relax.

• •

  ◊ Remember the healthiest time in your life. You were very healthy and you felt that you could do anything. Your body felt strong and alive. Your eyes were clear and bright. You knew that your bones and teeth were strong. You felt flexible and supple. You had lots of energy. You were free. Remember these good feelings.

Right now all your problems and concerns have disappeared. Let yourself experience this strong and secure feeling. There is nothing to be concerned about. Keep this wonderful feeling of good health. See a clear, beautiful green color coming into your body. Quietly and gently, watch this beautiful green color slowly fill your body. Think about your thyroid. Know that it is very strong and that it is functioning in perfect balance. Think about your digestive system and feel it getting stronger. All of your organs are acting in harmony with each other. The food you eat gives you the strength and energy you need. Your stomach and spleen are strong and relaxed. All your worries are gone now. There is only a warm, peaceful feeling filling you. With each breath, stress and tension are leaving you. Feel your circulation increasing. Your hands and feet are feeling warmer as your liver is becoming smooth and strong. Your blood is flowing easily throughout your body. From the top of your head through your torso, down your arms to your fingers and down your legs to your toes you experience the warmth that comes with a healthy circulatory system.

Let yourself experience this soft feeling traveling through your body. You can see the beauty that surrounds you. You are feeling more peaceful. Now think about your lung getting stronger. Feel your lung increasing in energy. Feel the air filling the entire cavity of your lung. When your lung has filled to its capacity, just let it leave your body gracefully, naturally. Your skin is getting clearer, smoother, fresher, younger looking. Your hair is healthy and shiny. You can feel your energy traveling through your meridians all the way down your body into your kidney and bladder. The water in your body flows evenly. You feel your kidney getting stronger. Your bones and teeth are strong and healthy. Your kidney is strong and helps you to pass out excess water from your body. You feel safe and strong. You have a beautiful feeling of balance, harmony, and health throughout your whole body. Now, feel your connection to the Universe. Take a deep breath in as you feel this connection. Breathe out as you open your eyes slowly. Keep this good feeling with you and remember it at any time.

CHAPTER 8
WEEK 4:
Making the Most of Your Healing Journey

*W*ELCOME to Week 4! Now how are you doing? This week can be a challenging one for many people. Don't stop doing what you're doing, and don't give up. Everything you've worked for is coming together. As your body begins to heal itself, it will make its own changes. This might be a good time to use your Healing Journal to explore these changes. Remember that the goal of the program is to heal the deep-down root cause of your excess weight. Be patient and be kind to yourself. You are doing excellent work.

Experiment with the foods on the list. Try out new recipes; be adventurous and combine these foods in interesting ways that suit your own tastes. All the items have been chosen for a healing purpose. They have not been selected because of their calorie count or their nutritional value, although naturally enough they are all good for you. The Dragon's Way, however, goes beyond the scientific and deals with Qi or vital energy. These foods are valuable for this program precisely because the essence, or "Qi," of each food helps strengthen and rebalance one of your five major organs. How do we know this? TCM practitioners discovered this information many centuries ago and have used it continuously to help millions and millions of people heal themselves. Although these foods offer great healing benefits, alone they are not powerful enough to help you address the root cause of your excess weight. They need the Qi-enhancing movements of The Dragon's Way.

This week you'll discover how your spleen/stomach partnership works and why maintaining this pair's balance and harmony is absolutely essential if you want to stay at a normal weight.

As in Week 3, this week may find you working hard to get through it, but tell yourself this is truly worth it because at last you are dealing with the root cause of your excess weight. Like some Dragon's Way participants, you may be in the midst of struggle or you may find yourself caught up in big changes. No matter what it is like for you, don't give up now. You are like a swimmer in the middle of the river. To go back means you must start all over again (if you ever do!). So continue to move forward and get to the other side.

The next seven days are a pivotal time as many individuals begin to experience a lot of changes both inside and out. Quite a few people finally see excess weight and inches begin to leave their bodies. Those who have already started to discard extra baggage often experience even deeper changes during Week 4.

Why do things begin to change now? As I have explained, your body's nature is to try and rebalance itself, to get to a state of health and harmony. All its systems have ingrained messages of self-regulation. But when it's been unbalanced for a while, it requires a lot of Qi to change. The goal of The Dragon's Way is to increase your storehouse of available Qi so that true healing can occur. The fact that you have been eating for healing and doing Qigong consistently for three weeks straight most definitely has helped increase your supply of Qi. Thus, your internal strength can now automatically bring your mind, body, and spirit into a more harmonious communication. When this happens, your body will function better and more efficiently. Once internal harmony begins to be restored, then your body can automatically (and naturally, I might add) drop excess pounds and inches.

There is an ancient Chinese saying: "To change the outside of yourself, you must begin from the inside." Given what you are experiencing, I know you can appreciate the meaning of this adage more fully.

Now I must warn you, not all change is comfortable or comes with a warm, fuzzy feeling. Deep healing comes with a price, and that price can be discomfort in the form of a runny nose, restlessness, a rash, or an unusual itch. Symptoms of healing transitions vary from person to person. Some people may experience a variety of these symptoms; others do not experience any such symptoms.

The most common reaction seems to be the itchiness. In describing this sensation, some people say that it feels like cobwebs on their face or body. Others describe it as a ticklish sensation under their skin that gently moves around to different parts of their body. For almost everyone, it's a feeling that comes and goes. Accompanying this itching is oftentimes a small rash that frequently appears behind the leg or at the elbow.

Both the itching and the rash are signs that your Qi is moving through the meridians, that your fat is beginning to "melt," or water is being released. It is also an indication of where Qi is beginning to free itself up. Because we are all unique, exactly how and where on the body a rash or itch occurs is also unique to every individual. As the "unstuck" Qi moves, over the course of several weeks, the symptoms can also move to other parts of your body. For example, an itchy rash behind the knees can indicate your kidney or bladder might be ridding itself of water weight that week; if the same symptoms occur around the rib cage, it can mean that your liver or gallbladder Qi is beginning to move. Once again, it might be helpful to write down in your Healing Journal where and when these changes occur and how you feel as they do.

As I said, some people experience a restlessness or a runny nose and other cold-like symptoms. If you are experiencing these or other minor discomforts, don't worry. And I ask you please to not try and suppress them! Many people believe this constellation of symptoms is caused by an allergy or cold, and fall back into old patterns of trying to block them with over-the-counter medication. Instead, I suggest that you turn to the self-healing practice of *Wu Ming* Meridian Therapy or try one of the various balancing recipes in this book, such as ginger tea.

The fourth week into The Dragon's Way, I broke out in big, itchy, red blotches. I thought, "It must be an allergic reaction to something." I was ready to take an antihistamine when I remembered that symptoms like these were caused by moving and changing Qi. It was at that moment I realized that The Dragon's Way was working, and I felt so motivated to go on!
SHOSHANA W., 35-YEAR-OLD SALESWOMAN

At this point in the program, it's time to concentrate on ways to increase and save your available Qi even more. An easy way to do this is each morning write down one way you can save Qi on that day. Some people do this right before they go to bed so that they're ready to implement their plan the following day. In Chapter 3, I gave you a few ways to conserve your Qi. Here are a few reminders and some new suggestions:

- Go to bed before midnight.
- Eat only warm foods. If you eat out at a business lunch, skip the ice water and ask for a cup of hot tea to begin your meal.
- Complete an unfinished task. This way you won't spend time or emotional Qi worrying about it.
- Practice moderation. For example, when you eat, really

try to feel when you're about 70 percent rather than 100 percent full.

- Practice, practice, practice Qigong. If you're standing at the copy machine or waiting in line at the store, very slowly and subtly do *The Dragon Kicks Forward* or *Backward* (#2 and #8). Don't worry, people may think you've been running and are just stretching your legs! Only you'll know that you're going beyond the physical to the energy level.

The Dragon's Way gives you the opportunity to take more control of yourself and your life—and particularly over the stress that overwhelms us so much of the time. Stress is everywhere. It can come from so many things—overwork, exams, worry, fear, traffic, and unresolved emotions. It can come from good things too, like having a new baby, getting married, landing a new job, getting a promotion, moving, and so much more. Externally, you know a lot of the signs of stress; you know that it can tighten your muscles, speed up your breathing, make your head pound. Internally, stress can wreak havoc on your body as well—on every tissue, nerve, and organ, and on your ability to maintain emotional balance.

So what do you do? First of all, pay attention to the power of stress. And second, do something about it. Here's one small suggestion that could make a big difference for you:

- Start your day at work by sitting quietly with your eyes closed for two to five minutes before you do anything (only 120 seconds). If you become nervous or stressed, take two to five minutes again and do the same thing. Just sit quietly with your eyes closed. Notice the difference this simple action makes.

- Try to find more time to slip in small meditations of two to five minutes during your day. For instance, if you commute by car, take a few minutes before turning on your engine. Or take two minutes when you park your car. Or when you get to

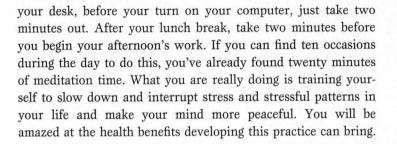

your desk, before your turn on your computer, just take two minutes out. After your lunch break, take two minutes before you begin your afternoon's work. If you can find ten occasions during the day to do this, you've already found twenty minutes of meditation time. What you are really doing is training yourself to slow down and interrupt stress and stressful patterns in your life and make your mind more peaceful. You will be amazed at the health benefits developing this practice can bring.

Now that you're at the halfway point in The Dragon's Way, you might want to re-read your Healing Journal. Many people find their Journal useful both during and after they finish The Dragon's Way. Keep your Journal by your bedside and write in it before you go to sleep or when you first wake up. Some people like to take a few minutes after they practice *Wu Ming* Meridian Therapy to add an entry. You don't have to write a lot. It can be just a few lines. What you write can be in prose or poetry; it can be questions or answers, observations or frustrations. You might even find that you want to draw something or create symbols. Listen to your intuition and let your energy, or Qi, flow through you at this time. You may be surprised at what you create. The physical experience of writing about, or taping, your positive changes, even small ones, can help imprint them in both your body and your mind. It's the difference between saving the information in a separate designated file on your computer or just putting it into your hard drive. Later, your Healing Journal and or tapes will make it easier to access the insights and data that you want to recall. You'll know right where you put them.

Participating in The Dragon's Way program was one of the best decisions I have ever made. It has impacted my life in ways I never thought possible. Prior to participating in the program, I suffered from severe migraine headaches that caused me to miss, on average, thirty days of work annually. I no longer suffer from these headaches, an improvement that

I can definitely attribute to this unique program. In addition, friends and coworkers have noticed a positive change in the ways I handle stress and in my overall approach to daily living. I am a much more even-tempered and happy person since I went through The Dragon's Way.

MONICA Y., 45-YEAR-OLD OFFICE MANAGER

QIGONG CAN HELP YOU GET PAST "THE WALL"

If you are experiencing mental and physical blockages, and feel frustrated by what you perceive as a lack of progress in your healing, once again, don't give up! Keep swimming across that river we talked about. Where are you ever going to find another program that considers the health and healing of your whole being? Where are you ever going to encounter a program that can address the root cause of your weight problems within an ancient medical system that has worked for literally billions of people? So, please stay on this path. You're doing fine, you just might have hit "the wall." I always tell people to turn to Qigong to help get past this wall. I cannot tell you enough how this is the most powerful healing tool I can teach you. It is so simple, but nothing works better to strengthen and increase your internal Qi than these ancient movements. The Chinese have been practicing them through the millennia. It is a very powerful secret we have kept to ourselves, until recently.

Now that you have been practicing *Wu Ming* Meridian Therapy Qigong movements for three weeks, I feel comfortable sharing with you some of their hidden power. I never like to tell people too much about them, because if you think a particular movement is good for your liver, you will *think* about that, rather than just *doing* the exercise. The aim of this practice is to become truly empty and open. I don't want you to set up your mind with a specific focus or fill it with visualizations. I definitely do not want your mind in control of this process or practice. This way, the body's Qi is allowed to follow its own course, doing what it needs to do to heal each individual at his or her own pace. Let me pass along to you a few secrets about how these energy movements can help you.

The Dragon's Toe Dance (#1) and *The Dragon's Twist* (#3) both cause Qi to move—in this case through the ankle, knee, and hip. That's good because most people gain weight in their hips. Through these two movements, an energy gate begins to open and Qi can then flow in these areas to help get rid of excess weight. Here's a tip. To get maximum benefit from *The Dragon's Toe Dance* (#1), try doing it both clockwise and counterclockwise. As you turn your leg outward, count 1, 2, 3, 4; 2, 2, 3, 4; 3, 2, 3, 4 and so on. Each complete circle is one count. Follow the directions in Chapter 3.

To help increase your Qi, try practicing the Qigong movements more often. If you only practice once a day, increase it to two times or do it once a day for a longer period. Another thing you can do is practice *The Dragon Stands Between Heaven and Earth* (#10) for at least ten minutes each day in addition to your regular practice. Or practice this posture intermittently throughout the day for a few minutes at a time. This remarkable posture is the most important of all. While the other movements clean out the internal "garbage" and move Qi through the meridians, *The Dragon Stands Between Heaven and Earth* is particularly powerful and can help strengthen your whole body and increase Qi.

HEALING WITH HEALING FOODS

As you will read later in this chapter about the spleen and stomach, you can accumulate a great deal of Qi through the food you eat. Many people ask me how much of each healing food they should consume. Because I am me and you are you, only you know the answer to that question.

I am quite fortunate because in China I had many masters who taught me about the healing power of food and the strength of my intuition to know what was right for me at any given time. I can only tell you that the more you believe, understand, and practice this concept, the stronger your intuition will become. Sure, you may make a few mistakes and pick out an overripe orange at your supermarket as you learn the power of your inner voice. But soon, your hand and heart will guide you, rather than your mind, which says, pick the reddest apple, which may, in fact, be rotten inside!

Therefore, I can only tell you that you will begin to know which healing food is right for you on any given day. What is good for you on Monday may not be what you need on Tuesday. Close your eyes and ask yourself, "What do I really feel like eating right now?" Certain smells may give you clues. Your mind may trick you and say, "chocolate cake." I say, "Go ahead and eat some chocolate cake." But, if you really want to change yourself, in time, you won't be fooled at all. You and your body will be able to have a very productive dialogue about what it wants and needs.

Other people also want to know if it is better to stir-fry, bake, or grill vegetables. It doesn't matter. I would like you to learn that it is the *essence* of that chosen food that has the healing power. Its DNA doesn't change with how it is cooked. So again, follow your intuition. If you're dying for stir-fried eggplant, then go ahead and eat it that way.

Another question people ask is: "Why red fruits?" I can answer that in one word: warmth. The essence of red fruits, no matter which fruit, is warm, and warmth can overcome dampness. For many overweight people, internal dampness is a common problem. So even though I cannot treat each of you individually reading this book, I can apply the same healing principles for everyone so that you can benefit from The Dragon's Way. I have selected red grapefruit over white, red apples and grapes over green, and so on. It's as simple as that.

FIVE MORE FOODS FOR HEALING

Let's take a closer look at five more foods for healing in The Dragon's Way.

Lotus Seed
A great food that can help your digestive system is the lotus seed. Because many people with excess weight have dampness in the stomach, the lotus seed, whose essence is warm, is very good for them. It can increase stomach Qi and help eliminate water. The lotus seed can be found in just about any Chinese grocery store. It can be cooked many different ways. You can make any kind of soup with it; you can cook it with chicken or other meats, and so on.

Chinese Red Dates
Another excellent food for the stomach, as well as the spleen, are Chinese red dates (not Western dates). They are used in TCM as herbs as well as food. With their warm essence, dates can aid the digestive system, alleviate sleeping disorders, improve blood deficiency (by increasing blood cells), and help the lung function more efficiently. Dates can also be used for a sweet soup with lotus seed. Or you can eat them raw by themselves.

Plum Tomatoes
The plum tomato is also a great healing food. It's good for the heart and stomach and supports their function. While other kinds of tomatoes are good for the stomach, I have chosen the plum tomato because of its unique ability to help the heart. Remember, I want to do as much as I can to help you in a

relatively short period of time. So stick with the plum tomato during the program. After The Dragon's Way, you can eat whatever kind of tomatoes you like.

Red Grapefruit

Some people find red grapefruit to be one of their favorite foods during The Dragon's Way. I'm not surprised because, with its warm essence, it is good for healing stomach function and can help the body pass out water through increased urination.

> *Each morning during The Dragon's Way I ate my roasted walnuts and red grapefruit. When I began, I thought, "Oh come on, this won't help me. I'll be continually hungry, just like I was on so many other diets." Then I realized, I wasn't hungry because of the Qigong. In fact, I was fine and processing food more efficiently than I ever had. About halfway through the program, I discovered how wonderful a little bit of honey and cinnamon tasted on top of red grapefruit. For me, this combination kept me full until lunchtime. And now that The Dragon's Way is over, I'm still eating the same breakfast!*
>
> PAT D., 48-YEAR-OLD INDEPENDENT RECORD PRODUCER

Walnuts

Walnuts are one of the most powerful foods that you can eat whether you are participating in The Dragon's Way or not. Walnuts, like Chinese red dates, are used in TCM as herbs as well as in foods. Their essence is warm, and they are so healing for the kidney and the large intestine. They can also help with lung problems and constipation, but are especially regarded in TCM for their ability to strengthen and increase kidney Qi, as well as improve memory.

TCM LESSON OF THE WEEK: THE SPLEEN, YOUR ENERGY GENERATOR

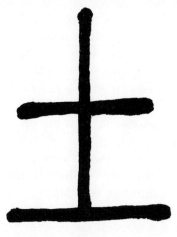

Earth

Dr. Li (1180 to 1251 B.C.) is considered the first physician in Chinese history to create the theory of the prominence of the spleen and its companion organ, the stomach. His wisdom can be reduced to one succinct sentence: "All human health problems are initially caused by a spleen/stomach dysfunction."

Why did he say that? Because proper functioning of the digestive system depends on the spleen which—with its partner, the stomach—is the body's main source of Qi after birth. Remember what I have told you about your checking account or Acquired Qi, the account from which the body's daily Qi expenditures should be drawn? You might say that your stomach and spleen are the main caretakers of that account.

Your stomach receives food and liquid and "rots and ripens" them, as TCM theory puts it. Your spleen then transforms this mixture into a refined essence called *"gu"* Qi. This food essence forms the foundation of your Qi and blood. Thus, the daily fuel and nourishment for your whole body depends on the spleen and stomach enjoying a healthy cooperative partnership. This is a lifetime linkage that you must keep strong to live a long life with vibrant health. If their function is weak, or if eating habits become poor—or both, as is often the case—the body will not be properly nourished. Then you can suffer from both deficient Qi and deficient blood. Also, according to TCM, if these organs are not functioning properly, you will definitely gain weight.

Look at the spleen's circle. You can see that:

- The spleen's partner organ is the stomach.
- Its element is earth.
- Its season is late summer. It's especially good to eat healing foods for the spleen during this time of the year.
- The spleen's direction is middle.
- The opening gate to the outside of the body is the mouth.
- The tissue it controls is the muscle.
- The emotions that can affect the spleen are overthinking, worry, and anxiety.
- Its environmental factor is dampness.
- The color related to spleen energy is yellow.
- The taste that goes directly to the spleen is sweet.

From the TCM perspective, here are some of the most common signs that indicate your spleen and stomach are not functioning properly:

1. Sleeping problems, such as insomnia
2. Bruising easily
3. Allergies
4. Cellulite
5. High cholesterol
6. Digestive problems
7. Lack of appetite
8. Fatigue
9. Muscle problems

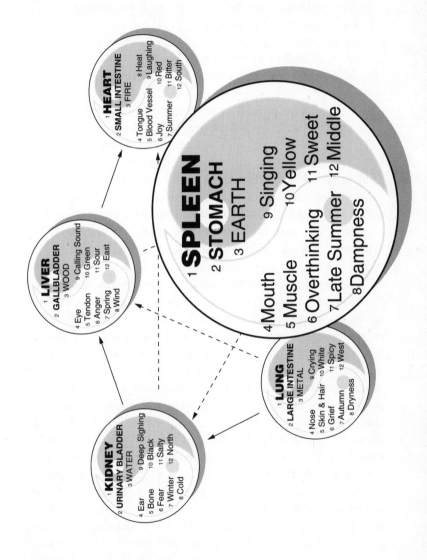

10. Menstrual bleeding problems, such as spotting
11. Migraine headaches
12. Anemia
13. Cold and/or sweaty hands and feet
14. Worry! Worry! Worry!

Why do these problems occur? It is the nature of spleen Qi to move upward: it sends food essence up to the lung for distribution and holds your body's organs and tissues in place. A weak spleen cannot perform these functions. Spleen problems tend to be ones of deficiency—the spleen seldom suffers from problems of excess. When your spleen Qi is so weak that it collapses instead of rises, certain organs can collapse as well, especially the stomach, intestines, uterus, and rectum. Other symptoms of weak, sinking Qi are diarrhea, fatigue, and blurred vision.

Your spleen has another important job. Besides transporting food essence, it also ferries fluids throughout the body. A weak spleen does not have the power to properly regulate all the fluids in your body. This is not good, since weak spleen function can lead to excessive dampness. We'll look at ways to recognize whether or not you have excess dampness. This is the organ that especially dislikes any kind of dampness because this environmental factor interferes with its work of transforming and transporting your nutritive essence. Poor spleen function can cause a range of digestive problems, including lack of appetite, poor digestion, loose stool or diarrhea, and abdominal distension. It can also cause you to retain water and gain weight.

Excess weight, of course, is probably the reason you're reading this book. So if you have trouble losing weight, the problem may be your spleen. Try this simple test to determine whether your spleen is not functioning well and your body is suffering from excess dampness. Look at your tongue. If it is fat, with a thick white coating, this is a signal that your body is unable to rid itself of excess water. Regular diet or weight loss programs and products as well as exercise cannot fix this internal root cause of excess weight. In fact, many overweight people don't understand that they are further damaging their spleen's ability to function by trying to diet in the first place. They are just weakening themselves further by denying themselves adequate and good nutrition. In fact, any diet that goes against the nature of any organ's function will ultimately cause more health problems later. You may lose weight in the short term, but you will upset your entire body's delicate balance in the long run.

As I said, the spleen moves liquids—including blood—through the body. It controls the flow of blood, how it flows, where it flows and how much blood should flow into a given body structure. The liver also relates to blood circulation, but its interest is only in storing blood and making sure it flows freely. It has no interest in controlling blood flow. It just delivers the blood. If the spleen has a problem, there will usually be conditions of internal bleeding. Women with poor spleen function may experience an abnormally long menstrual cycle or spotting between periods. A lot of menopausal women also suffer from frequent spotting and excessive bleeding. As you may know, hysterectomies are often offered as a solution to this problem. In fact, in the United States, one in three women will have had a hysterectomy by the time they are sixty years old. In my opinion, this is a procedure that is frequently unnecessary. According to TCM, the true root cause of excessive bleeding is not the uterus or ovaries, but deficient spleen Qi. Reviving spleen function with herbs and acupuncture can often relieve excess bleeding within a few days or a week or so.

The tone and elasticity of blood vessel walls is also the spleen's job. If the organ is too weak to perform this function, your blood vessel walls can become fragile and even collapse. This may cause bruising, varicose veins, and chronic bleeding. Fixing this problem means going to the source and helping the spleen regain its ability to function normally.

Before I end this chapter, I want to add some information about the stomach, which is the spleen's partner organ. TCM considers your stomach a bowel; that is, it fills up with food and water, digests and transforms these materials, then empties itself. TCM places tremendous importance on stomach Qi. While the kidney forms the energy foundation of the whole body, it is sufficient stomach Qi that gives each of the organs enough power to perform its job. You can see then that a deficiency of stomach Qi can lead to weakness in all of the organs. As we've seen, a properly functioning stomach working in cooperation with your spleen supports the daily activities of your body. According to TCM theory, whether or not your body can recover from illness or disease also depends on a strong spleen/stomach partnership.

From my experience, stomach problems—either of deficiency or excess—are always connected to liver function problems. Why? These two organs share a control relationship, and it's the liver's function to keep this relationship in balance. If the stomach suffers from a Qi deficiency, then naturally digestive problems will follow. Here are a few signs that will help you identify a stomach Qi deficiency:

- You feel relief from your stomach pains after you eat.
- You experience stomach bloating and loose stool.
- You have a fat tongue with a white coating.
- Your hands and feet always feel cold.
- You bruise easily.
- You are overweight.

Generally speaking, if your stomach pain goes away if you rest, massage it, or eat something warm, your condition is one of deficiency. In the case of a Qi deficiency, make sure you avoid cold food, cold fluids, raw vegetables, and excessive use of dairy products as much as possible. Stomach Qi deficiency can also cause hypoglycemia and migraine headaches. In this case, the migraine headache will usually occur across the front of the forehead, which is where the stomach meridians run. This Dragon's Way participant made big changes once she understood how the spleen/stomach partnership works.

Since I took this program, I have been eating better and have more energy than I've had in more than a decade. After repeatedly gaining and losing weight, I found that I couldn't take the weight off no matter what I did. I have a very hectic schedule and I eat erratically. I ate lots of salads and raw vegetables, thinking that these would keep me going and keep my weight in check. I was puzzled when my digestion got worse, I had constant stomach pains, I felt hungry and tired all the time, developed insomnia, and then a chronic yeast infection that made my life miserable. I was a mess of symptoms without an illness. All my doctors said I was fine, which of course was not true. This program educated me about how cold foods and foods with a cold essence were damaging my stomach function. I had never heard this information anywhere. First I stopped eating raw vegetables, then I started practicing Wu Ming *Meridian Therapy Qigong movements. I practiced twice a day because they made me feel terrific. They became the favorite part of my day. When I completed the program, my energy was really strong. My digestive problems went away for good and so did my stomach pains and insomnia. My yeast infection finally cleared up and I also lost eight pounds. My schedule no longer drains all of my stamina and I've become calmer and clearer.*

MEGAN N., 47-YEAR-OLD LAWYER

I'd like to emphasize to women readers that it is most important for you to understand that the stomach meridian runs up through the breast area where more than 50 percent of breast cancers are diagnosed. Keeping your stomach function healthy can help Qi flow freely through your stomach meridian, which, in turn, can help you prevent breast cancer from developing in this area. If you would like more information about how meridians relate to breast cancer, you can refer to our first book, *Traditional Chinese Medicine: A Woman's Guide to Healing from Breast Cancer* from Avon Books, or visit our Foundation's web site at www.breastcancer.com.

Some individuals, on the other hand, have a stomach that suffers from a condition of excess heat caused by liver Qi that stagnates in the stomach. They experience a different set of problems such as burping, rib and stomach distension, and stomach pain. Often they have a sour taste in their mouth (associated with the liver), or persistent bad breath. Their tongue will have a yellow or sometimes a red coating. They may even be continually constipated. If these conditions occur, it is important to treat the liver as well as the stomach; otherwise, the root cause of the problem remains. Often this excess heat comes from an internal source such as emotional imbalances like continually held anger and relentless stress. Excess heat can also result from external sources like eating too much fried or spicy food, and drinking too much alcohol. This condition also has the ability to cause heartburn, a migraine headache in the forehead, as well as temporomandibular joint (TMJ) syndrome. Gums that bleed or swell are also related to excess stomach heat. As you've seen, I usually ask participants in The Dragon's Way to avoid raw vegetables, but in this situation, raw vegetables can be useful. Celery, cucumbers, green peppers, any kind of lettuce, and radish can help relieve this condition. When this condition heals, it's important to return to the practice of eating only cooked vegetables and avoiding lots of salads.

Here are the foods in The Dragon's Way that are especially good for strengthening spleen and stomach function:

Chinese barley
Chinese red dates
Cinnamon

Ginger
Lotus seed
Papaya
Peanuts
Radishes—white or red

MY FINAL THOUGHTS FOR WEEK 4

Remember, this coming week is like being in the middle of a
river that you are swimming across. Here you are, right in the
middle. To go back is unsatisfactory. To go forward is hard
work. In fact, when people quit The Dragon's Way, it is often
at Week 4.

For you, I hope the only way is to go forward. You *can*
continue and cross the river successfully. I believe that there
are great rewards for you on the other side!

You are probably doing pretty well with *Wu Ming* Meridian
Therapy now. You may be using the breathing exercises or the
meditations during the day. Your outlook on food is changing
and hopefully your Eating for Healing has become an interesting
and enjoyable experience.

So have a peaceful week. Discover and honor your own
beautiful self. Don't let stress rule your life. Most of all, be
gentle and patient with yourself.

• •

WEEK 4: HELPFUL HINTS FOR GETTING THROUGH THE WEEK

- For relief from lower stomach pain, PMS, and difficulty
  urinating, heat together one to two bunches of chopped
  scallions and two to three tablespoons of wine or vinegar. Put the mixture in a cheesecloth or towel. You can
  steam or microwave this small "pillow" and apply it to
  the lower stomach like a hot water bottle or heating

pad. Be careful. You want to feel the heat, but don't burn yourself.

- As I've said before, avoid raw vegetables and even salad whenever possible during The Dragon's Way. Here's an easy way to cook your salad: Chop all your vegetables. Dice some fresh ginger root, fennel, and a little garlic. Mix them into your chopped vegetables. Bring several cups of water to a boil and immerse the vegetables in the boiling water for no longer than three minutes. Strain and add dressing. You will have eliminated the salad's cold essence, and now your body can save Qi in the digestive process.

CHAPTER 9
WEEK 5:
Going with the Flow

*C*ONGRATULATIONS. There are now only two weeks left in The Dragon's Way! By the fifth week, most people usually see major changes. Your body should be functioning much better than when you began the program four weeks ago. Many people lose inches during this week as their body's ability to regulate water, and even fat, starts to function again. If you've begun to experience changes during this week, it is because your organ systems are coming back online, so to speak. If you've suffered from being overweight for a long time, this is a good sign. You are reaching deep within to finally heal that root cause. And, if you've been overweight for so long, remember that this healing process will take time. There are no "quick fixes," just dedication and work. Unlike other programs, however, you are really addressing the source, not the symptom, of weight problems.

Again, be inventive. Try to stick with the Eating for Healing menu. Each of the recommended foods helps fix one of the organs responsible for maintaining normal weight, or they help increase Qi.

Most of all, continue your Qigong practice. By now, if you've practiced daily, you should look forward to working with these movements because of the clear, calm way they make you feel. Again, it's impossible for me to overemphasize how important they are. This is what makes The Dragon's Way work.

In this week, you will discover ancient wisdom that I believe you've never come across before. It relates to the lung. TCM uses the singular word "lung" and "kidney" to reflect its broader understanding of the physiological, psychological, emotional, and spiritual aspects that this holistic medical system perceives in each organ. In TCM, healthy lung function plays a critical role in maintaining normal weight. (Smokers pay particular attention to this chapter!)

I believe that if you have faithfully followed the Dragon's path, you have now begun to recognize what it feels like to awaken your healing ability. Perhaps it shows in the way you look, or the way others look at you. Your face will reflect your healing progress. You may feel a burst of exuberance at the beginning of the day. Or, you may simply have enough Qi to sail through your hectic schedule and not collapse in an exhausted heap at the end of the day.

How are you doing emotionally? By now, you have a good understanding of TCM and specifically The Five Element Theory (with all of its interconnected categories) to know that each of your organs has very clear and specific relationships with the others. You've also seen how each of these organs is affected by a specific emotional frequency or vibration.

As you've seen, whenever I describe a specific organ, I always tell you that each elemental circle also has its own emotion associated with it. Here's what they are:

Water (the kidney) is fear
Wood (the liver) is anger
Fire (the heart) is joy
Earth (the spleen) is overthinking, worry, anxiety
Metal (the lung) is sadness

TCM understands that different emotions, if excessive, can cause the function of different organs to fall out of balance. This is a most interesting TCM observation. If an illness is diagnosed as having its root cause in an unbalanced emotion, TCM says that the best way to treat it is to counter it with its corresponding or controlling emotion.

To show you what I mean, it would be helpful to study The Five Element Theory Chart again (page 133). Study each of the individual circles. In the circle relating to the liver, for example, you can see that the emotion associated with this organ is anger. Following the arrows, you see that the lung, which is sadness, controls the liver. Therefore, when my patients or students or Dragon's Way participants are feeling angry, I always tell them to go see a sad movie. Why? The answer lies with The Five Element Theory. Sadness, which is the lung's emotion, can control or fix anger—which is the liver's emotion!

Looking at the chart again, we also see that:

- Anger (the liver) controls overthinking (the stomach).
- Overthinking (the stomach) controls fear (the kidney).
- Fear (the kidney) controls happiness (the heart).
- And happiness (the heart) controls sadness (the lung).

Here are some interesting stories of how ancient TCM masters applied The Five Element Theory to treat physical conditions stemming from emotional causes.

FEAR FIXES EXCESSIVE HAPPINESS

In the Chinese culture as in many others, having a male child is extremely important. One old woman worried constantly about her son, who had three daughters but no male children. She worried about her family's ancestors and how the line could not continue without a male. She constantly prayed and made offerings at a nearby shrine for a male grandchild. One day, her son told her that his wife was pregnant again. During her daughter-in-law's pregnancy, the old woman prayed continually for a grandson. When she heard that the child was a male, she became elated—so happy that her line would continue. Her happiness was unbounded. It literally exploded within her. All of a sudden, the old woman lost all her strength; she became listless, and could not walk any great length or at a reasonable pace. Her son became alarmed and brought her to many different doctors and acupuncturists.

One day they visited a new doctor. The son went in first to explain his mother's condition, when and how it first started. The minute the doctor saw the old woman, he immediately approached her with a kindly but alarmed look. He came up to her, saying quite loudly, "Your son has described your serious condition. I do believe I must do surgery on your knee at the earliest opportunity. Please come closer so we can settle on a date now!"

The old woman looked at him in absolute fright for one split second, then she ran from the office as fast as she could. Her problem of excessive happiness was cured, and her ability to walk returned.

This doctor had used happiness' controlling emotion of fear to fix the problem that he had understood from the woman's son had stemmed from an emotional cause.

Here is a modern-day example of how this technique works.

ANGER RELIEVES WORRY

A patient of mine named Mary worried constantly. She was always thinking, thinking, thinking. According to The Five Element Theory, overthinking is associated with the stomach. So

I deliberately tried to make her experience anger (remember, anger, the emotion associated with the liver, controls worry, the spleen's emotion). Mary was always calling my office, worried about different health problems, especially her lack of appetite. So for a short time, I told my assistant to help her, but tell her I was not available. Not being able to talk directly to me made her very angry. After a few weeks, Mary came to my office and in front of everyone angrily told me that I was wrong for not calling her back personally. The very next day she came to see me and apologized for being so angry. She also wanted me to know that she was feeling much better and that she was surprised to report that her appetite had suddenly returned. That's when I told her that I had gotten her angry on purpose to relieve her overthinking. In my opinion, this was the best time-tested TCM way to deal with the root cause of her problem. Without understanding that the source of her stomach problem was an emotional one, Mary could have spent years looking for medical solutions.

TCM practitioners were using psychology many centuries before it was "discovered" by Western psychology. TCM has a sophisticated medical framework within which it can understand that emotional problems can indeed cause physical ones—such as the toll stress and anger take on peoples' lives and livers. That's why I continually urge participants who go through The Dragon's Way to use it as an opportunity to change their lives.

Here's an ancient story about the concept of "letting go" of stress and worry that you might find helpful.

A Buddhist master and his student were walking toward the river bank when they suddenly saw a young woman who was very distressed. This was somewhat of a problem because in their religion they were forbidden to look at, or even speak with, a woman. She, however, was deeply upset because she had to cross this river in order to continue her journey to reach her sick father. She begged the master and his student to help her get across the river. Very gently, the master picked her up and carried her through the shallow water and then put her down on the other side. He said goodbye and went on his way with the student.

Being a master, he could tell that his student was quite upset, even though the student was silent for the rest of their journey. Finally, that night as they were preparing for bed, he said to his student, "Is everything all right?" "No," the student exploded. "Everything is not all right! You spoke with a woman today and then carried her across the river. How could you do that? Our religion tells us that this is wrong." The monk replied, "Really, when did I do this?" "This morning, this morning!!" his student shouted, becoming more agitated. "Oh, this morning. Now I remember," said the master. "I already put her down, but you've been carrying her all day long."

QIGONG AND ITS REMARKABLE HEALING POWER

The Dragon's Way is an integrated program that combines energy movement and eating for healing. One complements the other. While each supports the other, Qigong is always the most powerful of the two. Combining these two things, you can see remarkable internal and external healing—including a change in your emotions. I know you are eager to learn what the other movements can do to help you in this process. Here are some more insights into this remarkable ancient healing art.

The Dragon Kicks Forward (#2) enables your stomach and your digestive system to improve. It also helps your spleen and stomach recover their ability to function, or perform their assigned tasks within the body, and become stronger. When you reach this level, your digestive system should perform very well. And, you should be able to eat any foods you want—even those to which you may have been allergic. Although TCM practitioners would never characterize it in this way, in Western terms, this Qigong movement has the ability to help improve your metabolism.

While *The Dragon Kicks Backward* (#8) seems similar to *The Dragon Kicks Forward* (#2), the two have very different functions and effects. Actually, *The Dragon Kicks Backward* is more like *Rocking the Baby Dragon* (#7), because these movements open two different energy gates that allow Qi to move freely up and down your spine. *The Dragon Kicks Backward* opens the basement door, so to speak, while *Rocking the Baby Dragon* opens the ceiling—that's why your Qi can flow more freely. Both movements can relieve back and neck pain. They can also help the body lose water by enabling the bladder to function more efficiently. In TCM, the kidney and the bladder are partner organs. Strengthening the bladder can provide tremendous benefits to the kidney and help you take off pounds and inches.

While practicing any of the Qigong movements, if you have a problem with your balance on the left side, most of the time it's because your liver is not functioning properly. In TCM theory, the liver governs the left side of the body; the lung governs the right side. I often repeat this to our participants: your physical liver (or lung) may be absolutely fine. It is the way it is functioning that is out of balance. A helpful analogy is to think of your body like a computer. The hardware is fine, but the software has a problem. A balance problem on the right side indicates a lung energy problem. A simple way to improve your balance is to keep your head level. When you practice Qigong, visualize a string emanating from the top of your head. Imagine that this string is pulling your whole body upward and gently holding your neck and head in a straight line. This will definitely help keep your spine straight.

Many of you spend your day in front of your computer or at a desk. If you feel achy and stiff after sitting for hours, stop what you're doing and take five minutes to practice *Rocking the Baby Dragon* (#7), followed by *The Dragon Kicks Backward* (#8).

And if you can, give yourself another three minutes and do *The Dragon Stands Between Heaven and Earth* (#10). You will be amazed at the effect these simple but powerful Qigong movements have on your neck and back pain. Not only that, but by taking the time out to destress yourself and treat yourself well, you'll become a happier, healthier, more productive worker.

MORE EATING FOR HEALING INFORMATION

Quite often, this is the week when people begin to say how sensitive their tastebuds have become. They can really distinguish the difference between fresh foods, processed foods, and foods with chemicals and additives. Foods that they thought they loved no longer taste the same. For instance, they may have loved potato chips before The Dragon's Way, and they may still. Yet, if they get a bag that's been sitting on the shelf too long, they can immediately taste if the chips have become stale or rancid. Many students tell me they could never have developed this skill without the program. If you continue to pay attention, this acute sensitivity can remain with you for the rest of your life. It will help you become aware of the foods your body needs at any given moment. It will also give you insight into when your intuition is saying "no," although your mind is saying "yes." Sensitivity to taste is all part of your newly developed skill to awaken your healing ability.

MORE SPECIAL FOODS THAT TCM PRESCRIBES FOR HEALING

Lily Bulb

TCM uses lily bulb to strengthen lung Qi. It can be incorporated as a food into your daily diet. You can create a delicious sweet soup by combining lily bulb with Chinese red dates and lotus seeds. You can find lily bulb in most Chinese supermarkets.

Peanuts

Peanuts are good for the spleen and stomach and are excellent for helping increase the volume of blood. These popular nuts are also good for helping produce milk in women who breast-feed. Avoid the oversalted kind.

Almonds

Here is another nut with healing properties. Almonds are good for improving lung function. Most Americans eat the large kind of almonds, which TCM calls sweet almonds. There is another kind called bitter almond, which has more healing benefit than the sweet ones. TCM uses bitter almond to help the lung relieve any kind of cough or function disorder relating to the lung.

Pears

Here is a remarkable fruit. Pears are particularly good for relieving heat in the lung or any kind of dry cough, skin problems, or constipation. The lung dislikes the condition of dryness; pear essence can bring soothing moisture into the lung. TCM prescribes pears (as well as kiwis) to relieve the kind of damaging internal heat produced by radiation or chemotherapy.

Fennel

Most people don't realize that fennel is a very powerful healing food. Usually white and with just its root, fennel is good for the liver, stomach, and kidney. Its warm essence can relieve conditions of cold in the body, particularly in the stomach and liver. I always recommend fennel to relieve menstrual pain and tell women to consume it before and after their periods. It can also help rid the body of stomach toxins. My students and Dragon's Way participants love to eat fennel sautéed!

Sesame Seeds

One of the foods for healing on the recommended list is sesame seeds, which come in black or white. Black sesame seeds are good for strengthening kidney Qi; white sesame seeds can improve the function of the lung. Both can help prevent hair loss and constipation.

Mint

Mint is an excellent herb for the lung, and therefore also good for helping to heal any kind of skin problems. Do you remember why? The skin is the "tissue" of the lung and as such is sensitive to the condition of this organ, as well as its partner organ, the large intestine. With its cool essence, mint helps relieve colds, headache and fever. It's also very good for promoting smooth liver function. Because its essence is very light, be sure to cook it—I prefer to boil—for a very short time. Two to three minutes should be enough.

THE TCM LESSON OF THE WEEK: THE LUNG: BREATHING THE BREATH OF LIFE

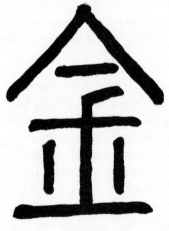

Metal

As we noted, TCM refers to the lung (as well as kidney) in the singular to reflect a holistic understanding of this organ that encompasses its physiological, psychological, and spiritual aspects. Your lung has many functions. From its high position in the chest, it governs both the formation of Qi—which occurs within the lung—as well as the distribution of Qi throughout the body. How does it do that? We've seen how your spleen (the mother of the lung) performs its job of sending the essence or energy of food upward to its child. What happens next is that inhaled air combines with this food essence in the lung. The lung then produces *"zong"* Qi (a kind of a master Qi), which becomes the basis for other types of Qi that are then sent out, like messengers, to nourish, moisten, warm, and protect your body. All of this happens, of course, in less than the blink of an eye. The lung, therefore, is considered to be the "manager" of Qi and nutrition.

This vital organ also plays a part in promoting the circulation of blood. While your heart controls your blood vessels, your lung helps create the energy to push blood through them. If your lung is weak, circulation will be poor, and your body will not be properly warmed and nourished. Symptoms of insufficient lung Qi include cough and shortness of breath, cold limbs and hands, sweating, and fatigue.

As I've said before, your lung is a key player when it comes to the body's metabolism of water. Two other organs—spleen and kidney—also have a role in water elimination. Each of these organs controls water in different parts of the body. In general, the lung controls water flow in the upper body. The spleen controls water in the middle body. And the kidney, naturally enough, controls water in the lower body. If you have a water retention problem, no matter what area, The Dragon's Way can really help your body regain its normal function because it specifically addresses the three water-controlling organs through Qigong and foods for healing.

One of the lung's functions is to direct your body's water downward to the kidney and urinary bladder for elimination. A weakened lung can cause urinary problems or water retention (if you tend to be overweight, it may be a lung function problem). And because your lung has a close energy relationship with the large intestine, constipation and diarrhea can also have their origins in poor lung function. Obviously, smoking can impair lung function. Smoking can also cause all kinds of skin problems, especially wrinkles, because it destroys healthy lung function and passes along this dysfunction to the lung's partner, the large intestine. It is the meridian of the large intestine that carries both Qi and nutrition to the wrinkle-prone areas of the face.

Now let's look at the lung's elemental circle in The Five Element Theory. You can see that:

- The lung's partner organ is the large intestine.
- Its element is metal.
- Its season is autumn. So it's especially good to eat healing foods for the lung during this time of the year.
- The lung's direction is west.
- The opening gate to the outside of the body is the nose.
- The tissue it controls is the skin and body hair. It's part of your lung's job as the manager of nutrition to send fluids to your skin to nourish and moisten it. Deficient lung Qi can manifest itself in dry, rough, itchy skin and dull, lifeless hair.
- The emotion that can affect the lung is sadness.
- Its environmental factor is dryness.
- The color related to lung energy is white.
- The taste that goes directly to the lung is spicy.

Here are common signs TCM recognizes that indicate your lung and large intestine are not functioning properly:

1. Asthma
2. Constipation
3. Diarrhea

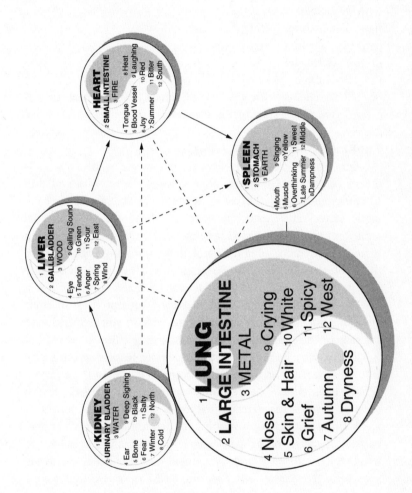

4. Skin problems of any kind such as acne, rashes, dry skin, rosacea, blemishes
5. Cough
6. Shortness of breath
7. Cold limbs and hands
8. Sweating
9. Fatigue
10. Problems with any loss of senses, like hearing, seeing, touching, smelling, and tasting

Luminous Skin and the Lung

One of the jobs of the lung is to disperse what TCM calls defensive or "*wei* Qi" to the area between the muscles and skin to warm and guard the body's surface. TCM believes that climatic factors such as wind, cold, and heat, etc., are external pathogens that can invade the body through the skin. Your skin is your first line of defense, and it is your lung's job to keep this protective mechanism working well. Weak lung Qi impairs this protective function and leaves your body vulnerable to a variety of problems, including increased susceptibility to colds and flu. This may be particularly applicable to you if you always get sick in the fall, the season that the lung rules.

That's why I always say that one way to conserve lung Qi is to dress warmly as the weather becomes cooler in the autumn. Windy days should be regarded as an enemy of good health because wind is the external pathogen with the most power to break through the body's first line of defense—the skin's energy barrier. Because other pathogens often attach themselves to wind, this is an easy and convenient way for them to invade your body. No matter what season, TCM views wind as a serious enemy, or disease-causing agent, to be vigilantly guarded against. So, if you can, stay inside on windy days. Certainly, if it's really windy, don't go jogging outside.

In addition to invading your body through the skin, external pathogens can also enter through your mouth and nose (the "opening" of the lung). Your lung is the only internal organ in direct contact with the exterior world. That's why it is extremely vulnerable to external pathogens. When your lung is invaded by cold, for instance, you may suffer from cold symptoms such as congestion, sneezing, and coughing. The TCM approach, to treating a cough caused by external cold is to try to expel it from the body. This contrasts with the Western approach, which tries to "kill" or suppress the cough with a variety of pills, syrups, and nasal decongestants.

Here's an interesting example of what can happen when a cough gets suppressed.

I have one patient who is a graphic designer in his late thirties. He came to me to try and cure a terrible skin problem on his hands and arms. The condition, which looked very bad, made everyone afraid to shake hands with him. If he handed over money, people were reluctant to take it. The fluid released by scratching his hands would often cause his girlfriend to have an allergic reaction. By the time I saw him, he had had this condition for more than ten years. He had been to many dermatologists and used many internal and external remedies. Nothing had helped.

At first, I used certain TCM treatments to address it as a usual skin condition. Although this helped somewhat, his skin condition continued to come and go. Then, I asked him if he could recall what happened in his life before the skin condition appeared. He then remembered having a severe cough for a few months for which antibiotics were prescribed. When his cough stopped, his hand started to develop a kind of eczema. He could actually remember the first site of this skin problem, which I recognized immediately as an area on the lung meridian. From my TCM background, I diagnosed this situation as one where the cough's energy was trying to break out of the body through its skin.

I told him that I was going to change his herbal formula, which would then change his internal energy. When this happened, I told him he might experience a cough. I told him not to worry about this cough because we would be allowing this old problem a way out of his body. As I knew he would, he began to experience the cough we talked about. In just a few weeks, though, his long-time skin problem began to show remarkable improvement. We continued this treatment for a few months. His hands and arms healed completely. This was about five years ago, and the problem has never returned. This case is a perfect example of how TCM theory can pinpoint the root cause of a difficult health problem. Without understanding the principles and theories of this ancient medicine, I must admit the treatment direction might seem a little strange.

Here's one of my favorite soups for relieving a dry cough:

Put a julienne pear, four to five almonds, the peel of one tangerine, and a little honey in three cups of water. Simmer slowly for about ten minutes. When finished, remove the tangerine rind and eat.

Before I started The Dragon's Way last fall, I got a terrible cough after walking around the city without a jacket. I made the pear soup for my cough and ate it at least twice a day for five days, and the cough disappeared. Then I started The Dragon's Way and soon five pounds disappeared!
MONIQUE V., 22-YEAR-OLD GRADUATE STUDENT

MY THOUGHTS FOR YOU FOR WEEK 5

TCM understands that the Universe is a circle and suggests we use this Universal shape to think about our lives and our bodies. Everything you can think of is part of the same circle of Qi or energy. Usually when we envision this shape, most of us first see a line drawing with nothing inside. Yet, this is not entirely accurate. The paradox of the circle is that it is both empty and full at the same time.

According to TCM, like everything on the outside of a circle, everything within is constantly changing. Therefore we, as humans, are constantly changing. Sometimes these ever-changing circles are referred to as cycles. Energy cycles happen throughout our lifetime. For females, energy cycles come every seven years; for men, it is every eight years.

If you follow TCM philosophy, your birth date is calculated by including the time from conception to birth as one year (even though it's really nine months). So, if you were born in 1960 and this year were 1989, according to TCM you would be thirty years old. The reason for this is that while you are in your mother's womb, you are physically on Earth and therefore accumulating and building your savings account—your Inborn Qi—while you are preparing for birth, the pinnacle of your Qi. At the end of each seven-or eight-year period, the body completes one internal energy circle. Whether you're a woman or a man, if you practice *Wu Ming* Meridian Therapy for the length of your cycle, you will see a tremendous difference in your life.

So remember to do what you can to keep your savings account Qi (kidney) strong by conserving and not using your Qi wastefully. And take the time to accumulate extra Qi in your checking account by eating for healing, doing the Qigong, and getting stress out of your life. Be serious about stress. Don't tolerate it for one minute longer. Be firm with yourself and those around you. Try to create a peaceful environment for yourself and those you love.

I had a patient who came to me for a problem that was rooted in a kidney deficiency. Although he faithfully followed the treatment plan I prescribed for him, there was no significant improvement. Then I learned that he worked the graveyard shift (11:00 P.M. to 7:00 A.M.). Following my suggestion, he was lucky enough to be able to have his shift changed to the swing shift (3:00 P.M. to 11:00 P.M.), and within a week he had an 80 percent improvement in his condition and continued to heal. Why? It takes at least twice as much Qi to perform tasks late at night as it does to perform the same tasks during the day. If you are one of the many people who work during the night, you need to give yourself extra care and attention. Practicing Qigong can help strengthen and increase your energy so that you don't overspend it.

This is not just a concept created for this program. This is ancient knowledge about natural law and how our bodies respond to it that TCM has applied for several thousand years.

So continue to practice *Wu Ming* Meridian Therapy every day this week and look for ways to save Qi, your most precious resource. Be careful not to squander it. And remember that food is a wonderful source of healing energy.

Most of all, be peaceful, build islands of calm into your day, and take good care of yourself.

••

WEEK 5: HELPFUL HINTS FOR GETTING THROUGH THE WEEK

- Here's a Qi-conserving tip: Keep your chest covered, especially in cold and windy weather. In the fall, make sure you're dressed warmly when you go out. Don't waste your Qi by defending yourself against the chill essence in the air.
- What about wrinkles and other signs of aging that show up in the skin, especially in the face? One of the benefits of taking estrogen is said to be that it reduces signs of aging, especially wrinkles, crow's feet, etc. TCM, however, sees skin condition relating not just to your age, but to the quality of lung Qi specifically, and the overall level of Qi generally.

  TCM believes that wherever there are wrinkles, there is an insufficient amount of nourishment and Qi to support muscle and skin health. Furthermore, with six major yang meridians beginning or ending in the face, having a facelift cuts through these vital energy pathways and can seriously damage them. It's like cutting off the roots of a tree. You may look better initially, but it's almost inevitable that some unwanted problems can develop later. This is why TCM's holistic approach concentrates primarily on reducing the signs of aging from the inside out. External treatment may offer some benefit, but there is nothing as powerful (or as attractive!) as letting good health shine from within.

- The only wrong way to practice is not to practice at all. So please keep up with your Qigong movements!

CHAPTER 10
WEEK 6:
You Too Can Be a Home Run King!

*W*EEK 6 is your own personal milestone. I hope you experience deep satisfaction and great happiness about learning how to heal yourself. I hope you have a good feeling knowing that you have awakened the power to help yourself change for good. And I truly hope you feel happy knowing that these changes are holistic and that you have changed, from the inside out. If you've been practicing *Wu Ming* Qigong movements faithfully, your energy level will most likely be higher than it has been in many years. Your ability to cope with the stresses of your life will have increased substantially. At last, your body, mind, and spirit are beginning to work as one holistic system. This is the beginning of true health.

During this final week you will learn about the heart, which TCM considers the king of all the organs. Many of the things you'll learn may be new to you; you might even find them amazing.

I like baseball, and I was very interested in the recent achievements of baseball great Mark McGwire. For the about-to-be graduates, I hope all of you feel that this was worth it. Maybe you feel as though you are Mark McGwire in that amazing winning season, stepping up to the plate with the bases loaded, knowing that it is possible, no probable, that you are going to hit a home run out of the park! If you've completed this program, I'm very proud of you, but even more important, I hope you are proud of yourself. If you didn't complete The Dragon's Way for any reason, you may choose to pursue this path again. This program is not a fad. These TCM principles and theories will be the same then as they are now. This book is like a treasure chest. It holds a lot of riches for you for self-healing whether it's today or tomorrow.

Most people who reach this point in The Dragon's Way have seen major improvements, both in their weight, inches reduced, and in health conditions that they never expected would change. As we discussed in the Introduction, during The Dragon's Way the average person takes off twelve pounds and about eight inches from her or his body. People also feel less bloated, are more energized and generally experience a greater sense of well being. Once internal harmony is restored, the body can automatically shed excess baggage and weight. Let's go back to our Chinese saying. I think it might have more meaning for you after all your hard work as you progress through this sixth week. Remember, "You cannot change the outside, only the inside." Here are some participants who were happy to share what they got out of The Dragon's Way:

For most of my life I was in good control of my weight. If I felt my pants were getting too tight, I could make some adjustments in how much I was eating, and I would feel fine after that. However, in recent years (maybe it's because I'm getting older) I had been about ten to fifteen pounds overweight and no matter what I did, I wasn't able to lose it. I'd go on a very-low-calorie, vegetarian-type diet. Then I'd try a fitness and exercise program, then I'd try an all-liquid diet, but basically, my weight would not budge. Then I started The Dragon's Way six weeks ago, and within the first two weeks, I lost ten pounds. It was a shock to me! I could even get into pants that I hadn't worn in five years. Plus, I had a lot more energy. Even now I feel real different. In fact, I feel like I felt ten years ago, and I thought this kind of feeling was gone forever!

JIM R., 36-YEAR-OLD MUSICIAN

Another participant wanted to share this story.

I started The Dragon's Way not so much to lose weight, but mainly because I was getting up in the morning and feeling really sluggish, with everything—from my back to my legs— hurting. My knees bothered me so much that I had to have surgery. And that's not all. Every time I ate, I had indigestion. I'd eat at the best restaurant in town, and I'd still feel terrible afterwards. In general, I felt like everything was going to pot. Then I started The Dragon's Way. By the fourth week, I started feeling better and losing weight. Now that I'm off the program, I'm not craving junk food and don't even want to drink soda or any of that stuff. When I feel that sluggish fog return, I do the Wu Ming Meridian Therapy, and I do feel better, and clearer. Also, my knees have stopped hurting for the first time in a long time, for which I am really grateful.

ANTHONY D., 38-YEAR-OLD DENTIST

If you are among the majority of people who have seen major improvements in your body, mind, and spirit, I have two words for you: DON'T STOP! Now the real deep healing begins. This is a lifelong process. So if you really want to achieve something extraordinary, as well as gain a deeper balance in your life, don't stop. It's great that during these five weeks you've changed your diet, followed the natural way, learned new and powerful Qi movements, and hopefully reduced the stress in your life. I can assure you that through this commitment and thorough work your body has been gently purged, gently energized, and gently rebalanced. What you've done is good, very good. But there's always more you can do. Inside you are still changing, so the most intelligent thing you can do for yourself is to continue.

If you are among those who have not seen as much positive results as you would have liked, it means your body needs more time. It does not mean the program doesn't work. Be patient, especially if you've been overweight for a long time or have a lot of weight to "give away." Your problem is deeper and requires more effort. You still haven't gotten to the root cause and healed it; your body needs longer to change. Perhaps your Qi is still stagnating or your organs are still not communicating with one another. At this point, you might find that a visit to a knowledgeable TCM practitioner or acupuncturist can help accelerate your healing. It might be that you could benefit from some classical herbal formulas to help strengthen your kidney, liver or lung function. Try to maintain your perspective: It's probably taken many years for your body to accumulate whatever problem it has, and six weeks is not enough time to make it completely better. But be honest with yourself. If you've followed The Dragon's Way, you should have seen improvements that you can point to. Take these as positive signs of healing.

As we conclude this week, I have the same two words for you: DON'T STOP! Keep going. If you do, chances are you won't revert to old patterns and your old lifestyle. These are the patterns that provided the ideal opportunity for weight gain or weight retention. You now have the healing tools to avoid these old patterns—especially the stress.

So, whether you're one of the people who have had great results with The Dragon's Way, or one of those who haven't seen the most benefits, you must motivate yourself to continue practicing what you've learned from TCM during these six weeks. If you only choose one way, the most important thing you can do is to continue Qigong practice. It is the most powerful healing tool I can teach you.

We've talked a lot about using your intuition to select and eat foods your body needs. Now I'd like to teach you another TCM secret. I want you to think about your body and ask yourself this question: At what time of day do my physical or mental issues appear or worsen?

For many people, problems arise or get worse at specific times of day. This has to do with the daily cycle of Qi among the twelve organs. TCM theory explains that Universal energy changes every two hours, and your body's meridian and organ energies respond to and match these changes. We are all woven into the Universe's web, so it makes sense that we are sensitive to and react to these changes. *In other words, each organ has a two-hour period when it is "on duty" or in charge of the body.* Our minds may not be aware of these Universal energy changes, but our bodies do respond to it.

During this particular time, the organ is like a traffic cop overseeing the flow and activities of the entire body. If that organ, or cop, is out to lunch or not functioning well, havoc can break loose with traffic jams as bothersome and serious as those on a thruway during rush hour!

TCM practitioners have understood this concept for millennia. They know when each organ is on duty, and use that information to diagnose a possible problem with that organ. For example, as the chart on the next page shows, the lung is in charge of the body from 3:00 to 5:00 A.M. If you find yourself waking up between these hours with any physical discomfort, including nightmares, it could be a sign that your lung Qi is weak or deficient. Likewise, if you are bothered by a symptom at 5:00 P.M., for example diarrhea, it could be a problem with your kidney Qi. In this instance, if you came to me with this symptom, I might treat your spleen (to deal with the diarrhea) with classical herbs, but I would also add something to strengthen your kidney Qi as well so that we could address the root problem.

DAILY CYCLE OF WHEN QI PEAKS

Lung	3:00 A.M.–5:00 A.M.
Large intestine	5:00 A.M.–7:00 A.M.
Spleen	7:00 A.M.–9:00 A.M.
Stomach	9:00 A.M.–11:00 A.M.
Heart	11:00 A.M.–1:00 P.M.
Small intestine	1:00 P.M.–3:00 P.M.
Bladder	3:00 P.M.–5:00 P.M.
Kidney	5:00 P.M.–7:00 P.M.
Pericardium	7:00 P.M.–9:00 P.M.
Triple warmer*	9:00 P.M.–11:00 P.M.
Gallbladder	11:00 P.M.–1:00 A.M.
Liver	1:00 A.M.–3:00 A.M.

*In TCM, the triple warmer is a meridian without a specific organ. It covers the areas of the upper body above the heart, the middle body from below the heart to the navel, and the lower body from the navel to the feet.

Here's one way I used The Daily Cycle of Qi to help a patient.

Not long ago, a well-dressed, spirited woman named Grace came to see me. She was fifty-one years old. For the last five years, Grace had worked the "graveyard" shift at a New York hospital. She sought me out because she had begun to experience bothersome menopausal symptoms, and didn't want to go on hormonal therapy. As I have already explained, by the time most women reach menopausal age, the stress and pressures of their lifestyle have caused insufficient kidney Qi and/or a liver dysfunction. As soon as Grace told me the hours she worked, I asked whether it was possible to change to a day shift. I said this because if you look at the chart, the liver's time to control the body is from 1:00 to 3:00 A.M. Luckily Grace was able to change her shift, and almost immediately her symptoms, which were related to a liver and kidney dysfunction, disappeared.

Remember last week's discussion about the lung? I told you

that your lung is like the assistant who carries out the orders of the chief executive; anything that requires movement depends upon your lung Qi functioning smoothly. Your lung is also the first organ to die. Because the lung is in control of all of the Qi you have built up after birth, when this critical organ expires, so do you.

As you see from the chart above, the lung's hours are from three to five o'clock in the morning. It is not surprising then that most hospital deaths are recorded during this time period. Individuals who are critically ill simply do not have enough lung Qi to go on. If they can weather this crucial time period, however, it means that their body has enough Qi or energy to fight another day to try and heal itself.

So my advice to you is use your intuition to become aware of possible problem signs by noting at what time of day the symptoms occur or worsen. Then, given what you now know about healing foods, choose the ones that can help heal the organ that might need an extra boost. You can also practice *The Dragon Stands Between Heaven and Earth* (#10) at the time your problem occurs.

QIGONG: WHY IS IT BETTER THAN EXERCISE?

Many people want to know what the difference between Qigong and physical exercise is. I tell them to look at it this way. Generally speaking, exercise can only make your physical body change. It is impossible to go beyond the physical without adding a practice like Qigong. There's no doubt that exercise can help you, and even fix your physical body and make it stronger. Physical exercise, especially if it's strenuous, cannot sustain you for a lifetime. Simpler things like Yoga, Taiji, Qigong, and swimming can.

Qigong, on the other hand, is about Qi or your life force, an invisible force that is every bit as real as gravity, earth magnetics, wind, and more. As such, its power is limitless. By working from the inside out, Qigong helps improve your body's function; it also balances your emotions and sharpens your intuition. It helps you become more calm naturally, and it makes you stronger, inside and out. We have covered a lot of this information already in Chapter 3 before The Dragon's Way Qigong movements. There are numerous studies in China on Qigong versus physical exercise. Now that you've been practicing for these past five weeks, you are much stronger. As we mentioned before, there are a lot of people who have built up their physical strength, but not their Qi or real life force. You have been doing this, and I hope you'll keep on doing it. Most of the people who can perform strenuous physical exercise or feats of physical endurance cannot stand for five minutes or more in the posture of *The Dragon Stands Between Heaven and Earth* (#10). Why? They simply do not have the skill to make their body, mind and spirit function as a whole system.

Qigong is different. I like to tell my students that everyone has a very special inheritance locked away inside of them. The potential is extraordinary for everyone. But most people have lost the access code. Qigong—by opening up your intuition and increasing your Qi—is the key to discovering this unlimited potential.

So if you want to experience something beyond feeling good and beyond the physical, continue to practice Qigong. With that in mind, let me share a few more things about the *Wu Ming* Meridian Therapy movements I have chosen for The Dragon's Way.

Three of the Qigong movements have similar purposes: with their "up and down" movements, they each give you an internal vacuuming, so to speak, and help stimulate your internal strength. They are: *The Dragon's Punch* (#4), *The Dragon Looks at His Tail* (#5), and *The Dragon Taps His Foot* (#6). All give you a great, whole body, internal cleaning. *The Dragon's Punch* (#4) can also help increase your balance.

Movement #9, *The Dragon Rises from the Ocean,* is one of the most ancient Qigong breathing practices. By breathing in fresh, new air and literally pushing out the old, used air, this movement helps control and revitalize your whole organ system. It also helps strengthen your kidney function and can help prevent your organs, like stomach, uterus, kidney, and others, from collapsing. Some participants have even reported that this movement has helped eliminate their hemorrhoids.

As you practice Qigong, don't think of it as exercises in a gym. This is not a competition to get in a certain number of reps. These movements are designed to increase the flow of Qi throughout your body. Just be mindful of the flow. Remember, with *Wu Ming* Meridian Therapy there are no special visualization or breathing techniques.

EATING FOR HEALING

For so many people, losing weight is about food, and *only* about food. When they begin the program, that's even true for the majority of participants in The Dragon's Way. That's why I continually repeat that we're focused on *healing the root cause of the weight problems and the stress that triggers them.* When you bring your body into balance, it will naturally shed the extra weight. But still, everyone wants to know about the food!

So for the benefit of all those people who are still thinking about food, I want to repeat that all the healing foods I've chosen for The Dragon's Way require very little Qi to digest. That's why complex carbohydrates and meats are eliminated from your Eating for Healing plan for these six weeks. Second, the foods are especially good for those organs which can cause excess weight and water: the liver, kidney, spleen/stomach, and lung.

During the six weeks of The Dragon's Way, our main goal has been to slow your body down so that it can function more efficiently. Think of your body like a battery that needs to be plugged in and recharged.

With this in mind, make sure during this last week (and for the rest of your life, for that matter) to eat a healthy breakfast before you leave home and before the energy of the day takes over. For most people, it's usually the one meal that you can definitely control. Try to eat slowly and calmly. If you have to rush out of your house, bring a few pieces of fruit with you, and then "steal" calm minutes at your desk or on the train or in your car to eat them. Taking a few minutes to do nothing but eat is a simple but powerful gift you can give to yourself.

FIVE MORE FOODS FOR HEALING

Red apples and red grapes

Two great fruits that are healing for your small intestine are red apples and red grapes. Their mild, warm essence helps the small intestine function more efficiently, making these red fruits excellent for improving metabolism.

Zucchini

Zucchini, which has a cool essence, is good for the stomach (and therefore the digestive system). This green or yellow vegetable can relieve constipation and bad breath. Zucchini is especially good for people with "stomach heat" problems.

Strawberries

TCM recommends strawberries as an excellent remedy for the gallbladder and its companion organ, the liver. This fruit can help the gallbladder function better, enabling it to pass more bile and digest fat more efficiently. Strawberries are also excellent for improving circulation and can help resolve sleeping problems.

Cinnamon

TCM tells us that one of the most important and ancient healing foods is cinnamon. With its warm essence, this wonderful spice is also a classical herb and an excellent remedy for both the stomach and kidney. It can help improve the digestive system, relieve menopausal symptoms, stomach pain, and frequent urination. This classical herb, which is studied in depth in schools of traditional Chinese medicine, can also help with arthritis pain.

THE TCM LESSON OF THE WEEK: THE HEART, KING OF THE ORGANS AND KEEPER OF THE SPIRIT

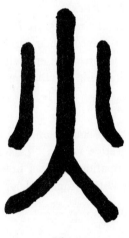

Fire

I always like to save the heart for the last lesson. This way I save the best for last.

In TCM, the heart is known as the king of the organs. Ancient TCM texts say: "If the king is happy, there is peace and harmony in the kingdom." While the kidney provides the power for the whole organ system, the heart provides its soul.

As you know by now, TCM says that every organ needs Qi to function. It also needs the right message or organizing force. This message comes from the heart. Your heart's job is to animate and inspire all the organs, maintain their proper function, and enable them to come together and act in concert, like one exquisite symphony. Your heart, as well as your liver, has a role in controlling the circulation of blood, but it also has another assignment: to control aspects of your mind and emotions.

To understand more about the king of the organs, let's go back to The Five Element Theory and look at the elemental circle of the heart. You can see that:

- The heart's partner organ is the small intestine.
- Its element is fire.
- Its season is summer.
- The heart's direction is south.
- The opening gate to the outside of the body is the tongue.
- The tissues it controls are blood vessels.
- The emotion that can affect the heart is joy.
- Its environmental factor is heat.
- The color related to heart energy is red.
- The taste that goes directly to the heart is bitter.

THE KING'S RELATIONSHIP WITH SOME OF ITS SISTER ORGANS

The Heart and the Kidney

More than any other organ, your heart must have strong kidney support (if you look at The Five Element Theory Chart, you'll see that the kidney controls the heart). Palpitations, for example, are a signal that your heart lacks the support of sufficient blood or Qi. If you experience palpitations, your heart is

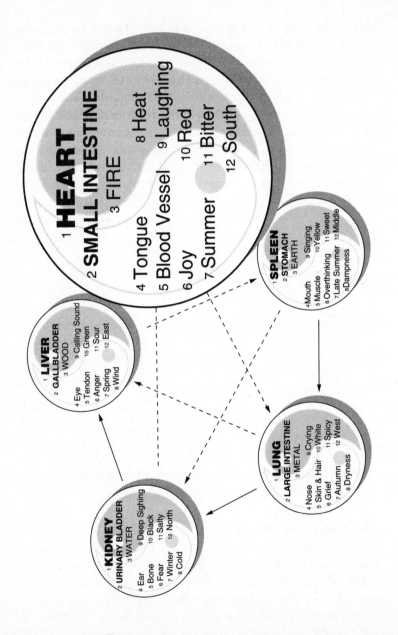

not getting enough blood. The problem is not insufficient blood supply; rather, TCM says that there isn't enough Qi or power to help keep blood flowing smoothly. Consequently, your heart must pump more forcefully to keep your blood moving. Strong Qi is essential to good circulation.

As you may know, in the West, heart disease is the leading cause of death among postmenopausal women. Why? From the TCM standpoint, menopausal women who develop heart disease also suffer from a kidney Qi deficiency. From what you now know about Inborn Qi, you undoubtedly recognize that older people, in general, are more susceptible to heart problems because their kidney Qi has naturally declined with age.

During our later years, the kidney has less Qi to draw on to do its proper job of cooling the heart or controlling its fire. Basically, your heart will overheat if your kidney is too weak to cool it down. According to TCM, you should look to your kidney to help your heart.

Your heart also controls body fluids. TCM says "perspiration is the liquid of the heart." If you perspire too much and too often, your heart may have a Qi deficiency problem, or conversely, excessive loss of fluid can cause a Qi or energy deficiency of the heart. This is why you may want to rethink your exercise routine, especially if it makes you perspire too much. By trying to improve your cardiovascular health, you may actually be impairing it.

Some signs that your heart may be overheated are:

1. Dry mouth
2. Thirst (especially at night)
3. Cold sores
4. Bright yellow urine
5. Skin breakouts
6. Nightmares
7. Poor digestion

Heart fire has the ability to affect your digestion because the heart and small intestine share a close energy connection. Therefore, an overheated heart can cause a fire in the small intestine—its partner organ—that plays an important role in absorbing nutrition from food. Too much heat in the small intestine creates an energy imbalance that can make your body feel uncomfortably full, or produce that infamous symptom—heartburn!

The Heart and the Liver

The heart also shares another close energy relationship with the liver, its "mother." In TCM theory, the three major organs having to do with blood are the heart, liver, and spleen: the heart controls blood circulation, the liver stores blood and regulates its flow, and the spleen creates both Qi and blood from the essence of food. The spleen also helps the liver by keeping blood flowing within the vessels. This intricate web of connections keeps your heart and consequently your whole body functioning smoothly. However, you know by now that if one organ isn't working properly, the whole system is compromised. For example, when your liver is overstressed, its Qi is pulled elsewhere and cannot support your heart's work.

CAUSE OF HEART PROBLEMS

The cause of some heart problems can be difficult to pinpoint. High blood pressure, for example, can be related to the heart, the kidney, or the stomach. As always in TCM, it is essential to identify which organ (or combination of organs) is the real troublemaker. But in the case of high blood pressure, the root cause is generally a combination of organs. High blood pressure is not a simple problem, because it comes from the functional disorder of all the organs. The entire body is out of balance. I've talked about the two types of Qi or energies in the body, yin and yang. The flow of each of these must follow its natural direction: yang Qi goes up, and yin Qi goes down. When you have high blood pressure, this doesn't happen. Too much Qi rises, where it gets stuck in the head. To treat high blood pressure, TCM will treat this upset in the imbalance of the body's energy system and try to get the whole body back in harmony.

High cholesterol and clogged arteries are other examples of function problems whose origins can reside in several organs. Most often, their root cause is in your liver. When any or all of the organs function poorly, your body gradually loses its self-regulating capabilities and falls out of balance. (Likewise, when your body is well, it manages cholesterol levels very nicely and keeps your arteries open.) This is true even if the organs themselves are fine physically. The body then becomes inefficient and sluggish. Substances such as fat, water, and toxins tend to accumulate. It's vital, at this point, to identify why your body is falling out of harmony. In other words, TCM will still search for the root cause, rather than just treat its symptoms.

Complex problems such as high blood pressure or high cholesterol do not receive disease-specific treatment from TCM. In fact, TCM does not even categorize these problems in Western medical terms. As you've learned by now, a good TCM doctor will analyze a patient's individual symptoms; then, diagnosis and treatment will focus on the organs determined to be the root cause. TCM does not separate a patient from his or her symptoms; it views the person as an integrated whole. It always looks at the larger picture of the condition of the body's energy system, as well as its relationship with the Universe. Over the millennia, TCM has utilized a vast body of experience and knowledge to bring a body in balance so that it can heal itself.

THE HEART AS KEEPER OF THE SPIRIT

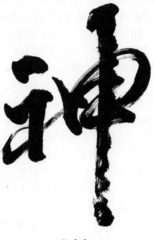

Spirit

As king of all organs, the heart, says TCM, houses the *Shen,* or spirit. It also considers your heart to be the ruler of all mental activities. When TCM speaks of the mind, it has a broader meaning than that in the West. It includes aspects of consciousness; intelligence and thinking; memory and sleep; emotions; and various aspects of the soul. In TCM's view, most mental and sleep problems can be traced straight to the source—unbalanced heart Qi.

Therefore, if your heart is weak or overheated as described earlier, or if it is not supplied with enough blood, your spirit cannot rest peacefully in its domain—the heart. If you've been stressed out or unhappy (at your excess weight, for example), I think you will recognize these feelings.

Undoubtedly you've experienced a time when your whole body feels uneasy and restless, your thinking becomes cloudy or fuzzy, and your memory is poor. Insomnia and nightmares may even occur. For instance, have you ever had a night when your mind seems to float, or worse, to race? Many of my patients talk about their mind "racing" at night when they are trying desperately to get to sleep. Do you ever feel like you are asleep, yet you're aware of being awake at the same time? For ages, TCM has viewed this condition as an indication that the heart is unable to "house" its *Shen,* or spirit. If you want to feel calm, think clearly, and sleep soundly, you must take care of your heart. Above all, if you can keep your heart in a joyful, peaceful state, you can also help reduce the effect of stress on the all-important liver. Why? Because this way the "child" can please its "mother."

TAKING CARE OF YOUR HEART

What can you do to take care of your heart? First, it is helpful to understand that the organ itself has powers and ability far beyond its physical structure. Think about how powerful your heart is and how strong its potential for unconditional love is. You know, real love comes from your heart, not your mind. Our most difficult struggle is between the heart and the mind. Although they may seem very similar, they are completely different. Your mind does your thinking, your heart handles your feelings, and they both try to guide us. That's why there's a continual struggle.

One of the purposes of our Qigong practice is to help open your heart, and thereby strengthen your intuition. In Eastern philosophy, many texts talk about meditation and emptying the mind. When the mind is empty, the heart can take a rest. It can conserve the heart's spirit, as well as its physical Qi. If your mind is always in motion, your spirit will be in motion as well. When your mind is empty, your heart can truly open. If you can reach this state, then unconditional love and forgiveness can enter. You can forget the past and move on. Enormous burdens that we carry can dissolve this way. When a heart offers unconditional love, it can reach infinity. Love is the most powerful way we can nurture and heal this precious organ. Smiling (a real smile) and being happy may sound too easy, but this time-tested wisdom brings us a simple truth.

In almost every Dragon's Way program that I run, someone always asks me if TCM has a special magic formula, pill, exercise or program to reduce wrinkles and maintain a youthful appearance. My answer is yes, and the good news is I can pass it along to them for free! The secret is—smiling from the heart. Smiling can nurture your heart and keep it forever young. In fact, TCM, along with many meditation systems, considers smiling from your heart the best cardiovascular activity you can practice. While this is a serious statement, I like to make a joke in The Dragon's Way. I tell my participants if you can reach this level, you can donate your treadmill to charity.

Here's an easy, yet at the same time very difficult, ancient smiling exercise:

Face the mirror and smile at yourself—really smile at yourself—from your heart. This is a very difficult practice for most people. Smiling deeply from your heart—not just a fake smile— actually has a physical effect. It will help make blood and Qi flow throughout your whole body. When you've mastered this practice, then try smiling at others from your heart.

We know that smiling and laughter can create emotional Qi and propel it through the body. This helps heal the heart; it's much more effective than physical exercise. TCM understands that it can cause the heart's spirit, as well as its physical structure, to change.

It's interesting to see how many phrases relating to the true power of the heart are used unconsciously in Western society. I'm sure you're familiar with many of them. For example, we say "You broke my heart." Is your physical heart really broken? No, but if you've ever had your heart broken, you know its spirit has been deeply wounded or affected. When we say "You're in my heart," does this mean that your whole body is in someone else's heart? No. It means that you carry their spirit with you. Even the popular song from the movie *Titanic* is titled "My Heart Will Go On," not "My Mind Will Go On." It reflects the concept that the heart's spirit lives on with its memories even though the body may perish. Other expressions? "I'm telling this to you from my heart"; "My heart is in the right place"; and "I love you with all my heart." To replace these phrases with the word "mind" simply won't work.

Here are the foods I've chosen for The Dragon's Way that are especially good for the heart. The energy essence or healing Qi of each of these foods is sent by the lung directly to the heart, where they can help strengthen or heal this organ:

- Broccoli
- Broccoli rabe
- Plum tomatoes
- Watermelon

MY FINAL THOUGHTS FOR YOU THIS WEEK

As you work through this final week, try to *feel* the difference between where you are today and where you were at the beginning of The Dragon's Way. Wherever your starting point was, I'm sure you intuitively know you have made a quantum leap from then to now. I want you to really *feel* the difference in your body. Our society makes us so busy that we're forced to continually use our minds and ignore the signals our body sends us. You are different now. Feel this difference. The Dragon's Way has already helped you recall this special gift. Don't let it slip away again.

In your Qigong practice, allow your heart to open. When you're too rigid, there's no space for the heart to work its magic. When there's emptiness, there is a vast space for healing. The highest level of Qigong is about training the heart. The mind must be empty. When we can totally empty the mind, then the heart can open. Allow yourself this life-giving freedom. Allow forgiveness and happiness to enter. Continue to make entries in your Healing Journal. After this week is over, you may want to set an evening aside and review what you've written (or drawn) during these past six weeks. I believe you will find a lot of interesting things in your Healing Journal that will help you with your healing progress.

Our final week of The Dragon's Way focuses on the king of the organs, and you should try and work at making your heart change. In other words, don't be afraid to step up to the plate and hit that home run!

So have a peaceful week. Congratulate yourself at the conclusion of the program and reward yourself for having the intuition to be drawn to this ancient healing wisdom. Most of all, look forward to your new life.

• •

WEEK 6: HELPFUL HINTS FOR GETTING THROUGH THE WEEK

- What causes the heart to change? It's not by "thinking things through"; it's by quieting your mind. Next time, figure something out by looking at beautiful things—like a sunset.
- Your whole face is related to your heart. Your face is the "freezer" of your emotions. If you can keep your emotions balanced and happy, then your face will reflect this special state. You may not think it, but your deepest feelings show on your face. If you change your face, you will change your heart as well. If you have a change of heart, your face will also change. This is nature's way.
- Just smile. A true smile will come from your heart.
- Try not to take yourself too seriously this week (and from now on).
- Follow your heart's path by realizing you cannot "control" anyone's action. The only thing you have control over is

your own reaction. Remember, action and reaction are an inseparable pair—much like yin and yang energies, or even Qi and blood. Whatever action is taken, there will always be a reaction and the reaction may not be to your liking. So accept the actions of others without attaching yourself to them. Learn to let things go.

- Continue to be patient, but act firmly. Think of an eagle when it soars from above to catch a fish. If she misses, does she panic or get depressed? No, she continues and patiently waits for the next chance, the next opportunity. In fact, she will continue to wait until the timing is just right. This is known as the Way of the Tao. Look at the way of the animals—they have a number of great lessons for us.

At the end of the sixth week, stop and take some time to fill out TCM Checklist II below. Afterwards compare your responses to the same TCM Checklist I that you filled out at the beginning of Week 1. Most people notice that their responses to TCM Checklist II are quite different than they were six weeks ago. All the progress you see is real. Your Dragon's Way journey has helped you deal with the root cause of your weight problem. Congratulate yourself. You are really changing from the inside out. After these six weeks, many participants have taken off twelve pounds and eight inches (and more), but most of all they feel much healthier, stronger and better able to cope with stress. I believe you do too.

• •

THE DRAGON'S WAY CHECKLIST

Your responses to the following questions will help you to objectify your progress. After you fill out this checklist, compare it to the one you filled out in Week 1 so you can see how far you've come over the six weeks of The Dragon's Way program.

Symptom	No symptom	Mild	Moderate	Severe
Fatigue	___	___	___	___
Dizziness	___	___	___	___
Palpitations	___	___	___	___
Night sweats	___	___	___	___
Shortness of breath	___	___	___	___
Chest pain	___	___	___	___
Back pain	___	___	___	___
Muscle tension	___	___	___	___
Loss of appetite	___	___	___	___
Abdominal distension	___	___	___	___
Headache	___	___	___	___
Stomachache	___	___	___	___
Diarrhea	___	___	___	___
Constipation	___	___	___	___
Skin rash	___	___	___	___
Dry mouth	___	___	___	___
Insomnia	___	___	___	___
Racing heart	___	___	___	___
Bone pain	___	___	___	___
Joint pain	___	___	___	___
Upset stomach or nausea	___	___	___	___
Sweaty hands	___	___	___	___
Difficulty sleeping	___	___	___	___
Irritability or restlessness	___	___	___	___
Depression	___	___	___	___

Symptom	No symptom	Mild	Moderate	Severe
Nightmares	_____	_____	_____	_____
Nervousness	_____	_____	_____	_____
Angry moods	_____	_____	_____	_____
Worrying	_____	_____	_____	_____
Loss of sexual interest	_____	_____	_____	_____
Forgetting information	_____	_____	_____	_____
Frequent urination	_____	_____	_____	_____
Cold hands and feet	_____	_____	_____	_____
Heartburn	_____	_____	_____	_____
Vaginal discharge	_____	_____	_____	_____
Irregular menses	_____	_____	_____	_____
Hot flashes	_____	_____	_____	_____

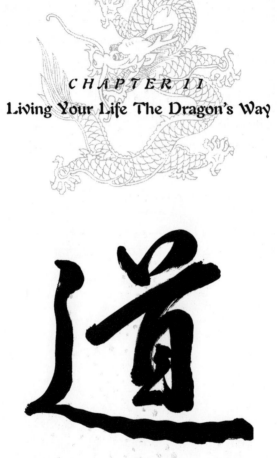

CHAPTER 11
Living Your Life The Dragon's Way

Tao

*A*τ the final class of The Dragon's Way, everyone has the same question: "What should I do now that the program is over?" My answer is that the program is never over and now that they have reawakened their own healing ability, they are ready to begin another phase of their healing journey. The skills and knowledge they have acquired is something they can use for the rest of their lives. Restoring and maintaining true harmony within the body and between the body and the Universe is not a one-day, nor a six-week, project. The Dragon's Way is a unique beginning but is, in reality, a lifetime's worth of work. The Dragon's Way is forever, as I hope your daily Qigong practice will be.

For a month and one-half now, you have been learning how to take care of yourself in new ways. You have been thinking differently about food and developing a new relationship with it. You have been choosing foods that will harmonize with your body and assist you energetically. You have learned that Eating for Healing is the way to use food as a medicine to help make profound changes. At the beginning of The Dragon's Way, you may have thought of this program as just another diet plan. But by now, you understand that it is something much deeper, something more lasting. Of course you may have taken off pounds and inches, but much more important, you have regained your life and health. Here's a perspective from one of The Dragon's Way graduates:

I had watched my weight slowly increase since my mid-forties. I dismissed all the rest of my physical complaints to being in my fifties and menopausal. I came to The Dragon's Way thinking that I would go on a "different diet" and "lose some of the weight." My first surprise was that this wasn't a diet. I soon realized that using this term limited the program to something much smaller than it is. The more I practiced the principles of Eating for Healing, the more I understood why diets never had long-term results. I didn't expect that practicing Wu Ming *Meridian Therapy and applying the principles of TCM would relieve my shortness of breath, eliminate my headaches and stomach pain, and give me the ability to cope with stress with greater calm. As these symptoms decreased, my nervousness and irritability also vanished. At the end of the program I felt great! I lost twenty-one pounds—more than I expected to lose in six weeks.*

I have more energy and my entire way of thinking about food and health has changed totally.
                                    MELANIE S., 53-YEAR-OLD SECRETARY

One of the major complaints of the modern world is that there is not enough energy. Now you really know about energy. You know about the real Qi of the Universe that makes everything move and flow. You have some real knowledge about Qi or energy—how to increase it and how to maintain it. *Wu Ming* Meridian Therapy is something you can use for the rest of your life to ensure greater health and vitality.

During The Dragon's Way, you have learned a whole new way to view your body, and about the interrelationship of your body, mind, emotions, and spirit. In other words, you have been learning to relate to yourself as an integrated whole. These six weeks may have brought tremendous change for many of you. Look how far you've come.

While you have undoubtedly been focused on shedding weight throughout The Dragon's Way, many other changes were taking place that were not necessarily as apparent to you. That is one reason I asked you to fill out the checklists so you could see for yourself the differences before and after the six weeks. As you can see, many things were happening while you weren't looking!

If you ate the healing foods and practiced Qigong, your body has begun the process of deep change, but it needs time to learn to rebuild and refunction. You did not wake up one morning with ten, twenty, thirty, or more pounds of excess weight. The extra pounds and other symptoms of imbalance of your internal organ systems happened over time, and you can heal the imbalances over time as well. If you were able to rid yourself of excess baggage during these six weeks, it is a sign that your digestive system is healing and that your ability to cope with stress is increasing.

If you have practiced the ideas and techniques presented here through all six weeks, consider yourself a graduate of The

Dragon's Way! But please don't stop practicing what you've learned. Now more than ever, it's vital for you to take this knowledge one step further.

While the formal program is over, the processing of Qi that you have initiated is not yet completed. Don't give yourself the message, "Oh, I'm done. I'm so good. I lost such and such amount of weight. I had these different health changes. Now it is over." *Health is not a destination; it is a way of life.* Tell yourself that The Dragon's Way is just beginning. You can gradually eat other foods. You can now add other things back into your eating plan. Don't deprive yourself of things you really love to eat, but notice how your body now reacts to them. The real benefit is not what you can do in six weeks, but what you can do for the rest of your life. You have literally awakened your self-healing ability. Be smart and nurture it so it doesn't go right back to sleep, or slip away forever.

Some of you who have achieved a certain level of healing might find that as time goes on you have hit a plateau. Be patient. Your body may need a rest. Even if you have not taken off very much weight or inches in these initial weeks, if you have been practicing the *Wu Ming* Meridian Therapy and Eating for Energy, your internal systems are definitely getting stronger. This is when you must trust yourself more and keep practicing so that you'll be prepared for the next breakthrough. Be patient and, most of all, do not start worrying. Worrying affects your spleen and your stomach, and it could put you back into a cycle of gaining weight.

Dr. Lu really captured my attention when he said "It is 100 percent your life." This simple statement underscored everything I learned about the self-healing nature of the body. I understood that I was being presented with the knowledge and tools to deeply develop my ability to be balanced, whole and healthy. I realized that no one was coming to save me but myself. I finally realized that I had the power to change myself at the most profound level. Now diet programs, pills, supple-

ments—all the externals that I used to believe would solve my weight problems—seemed small in comparison to what I know. Over the term of the program, I broke years of bad habits and now feel more aware of my body's needs. My energy has increased incredibly. I am astonished by the results I have had in only six weeks of Eating for Healing and practicing the Wu Ming Meridian Therapy. My weekly migraines have been reduced to one time this month. My menstrual symptoms are greatly alleviated; I am not depressed; my circulation is better; my memory has returned; and my bloated feeling and nightmares have left. All of this and I lost ten pounds.

VALERIE D., 50-YEAR-OLD SUPERVISOR

PRACTICAL ADVICE ABOUT EATING FOR HEALING

It's most important to remember not to slip back where you were before you started The Dragon's Way. You now know that Eating for Healing means more than just consuming the foods on a recommended list. You have come to understand the healing power of foods, their essences and which organs they can heal. Chances are, from now on, each time you put something in your mouth, you will actually stop and think about these things you've learned (you may make different choices, but you'll still think about the healing DNA of what you eat). When you go to the grocery store, chances are you will be excited about using your newly reenergized intuition to select and purchase food. Listen carefully to what your body tells you. What foods would you like to bring back? What foods would you like to taste again? How do you feel when you eat them? How much of them do you want?

As a graduate of The Dragon's Way, you are now free to eat meat, dairy, sweets, and hard carbohydrates. You can go back to drinking a glass of wine now and then. But with this new "diploma" also comes new knowledge and new responsibilities. So from now on, I hope you will give yourself that moment to pause and remember what you already know: you have intuitive power to eat for healing.

There is an ancient Chinese saying that tells us, "When you have more Qi, you won't feel hungry." The corollary is also true: if you don't have enough Qi, you will feel hungry. Therefore, if after The Dragon's Way you feel pangs of hunger, chances are your Qi is still not as strong as it needs to be for your life's activities. So what should you do? You should continue to build up your Qi through healing foods and, of course, by practicing the Qigong movements.

One of the easiest things is to eat foods from the Recommended Foods List for three or four days each month to give your body a good cleaning and rest. Think of it as your thousand-mile tune-up.

If you are among those people who did not shed enough weight or lose enough inches this time around, give your body more time. Your problem is deeper. If this is you, it would be best for you to continue with the Recommended Foods for another six weeks. It's not necessary to do this right away. Give yourself a few weeks in between, then go back to the program. Other people wait a few months to see how well they are doing. Many decide to go through another six-week cycle, while others do it for three. You know your body, and you know what it needs.

WU MING MERIDIAN THERAPY: A GIFT FOR LIFE

As I've said many times during these last six weeks, the most powerful healing tool I have taught you is the *Wu Ming* Meridian Therapy. If you do these Qigong energy movements regularly, I believe you will have enough Qi; and you *will* keep the excess weight and baggage off. But the key, of course, is practice.

You know, each day, most of us take a shower to wash our external bodies. How do you feel when you miss a day? Not as fresh as you would like to feel, right? That's how I feel if I miss a day of practice. I always tell people to think of Qigong as an internal shower, where each day you give yourself a good internal scrubbing and rinse—without it, your Qi can get clogged and you can feel not very fresh inside. With it, you clean out your emotional and digestive systems, recharge your Qi, and help your body and spirit soar. Take this unique gift of a lifetime and smile at yourself every day from your heart. You have awakened something special—the gift of self-healing!

THE POWER OF THE DANCE

So many people want to know the same thing: How do the ten Qigong movements help someone discard weight and reduce inches? How can they do this without strenuous exercise? How do they make me look and feel this firm without going to the gym? Think of them as a single, flowing dance. In the first act when you are just learning them, you, the dancer, are a mishmash of frenetic energy, but by the finale, you are a perfect flow of powerfully balanced Qi. Let me explain further:

In Act I, with the first movement—*The Dragon's Toe Dance* (#1)—you start to free the Qi in the lower half of your body— moving it gently around as you rotate your ankles, knees, and hips. Then, with *The Dragon Kicks Forward* (#2), you massage your liver—the organ which receives the brunt of our relentless stress. This movement also helps your stomach and your digestive system function better. Then, *The Dragon Twists* (#3) helps stimulate Qi in the six meridians that run through the leg and connect with the upper body.

In Act II, your Qi is now flowing more freely; it's time for an internal vacuuming and for moving the stale, or in some cases stagnating, Qi out of your upper body with *The Dragon's Punch* (#4) and *The Dragon Looks at Its Tail* (#5). The next Qigong movement—*The Dragon Taps Its Foot* (#6)—does the same for the lower part of your body.

How then does this stale energy get released? You accomplish this in Act IV with *Rocking the Baby Dragon* (#7) and *The Dragon Kicks Backward* (#8). These movements open two different energy gates, allowing Qi to move freely up and down your spine. *The Dragon Kicks Backward* opens the basement door, while *Rocking the Baby Dragon* opens the ceiling, allowing the stale Qi to be liberated and the strong, remaining Qi to flow freely.

What next? As you approach the finale, you take in more fresh Qi from the Universe and, once again, push out the stale, useless Qi with *The Dragon Rises from the Ocean* (#9). This very ancient movement helps control and revitalize your whole organ system, particularly your kidney, where your energy savings account is stored. And then comes the finale—with all this magnificent new Qi, your body needs to quietly gather itself into a state of harmony and balance, with *The Dragon Stands Between Heaven and Earth* (#10).

A beautiful performance, wouldn't you say?

SOME REMINDERS ABOUT YOUR QIGONG PRACTICE

For optimal benefit, it is best to practice the *Wu Ming* Meridian Therapy about forty minutes a day—twenty minutes in the morning and twenty minutes in the evening. Practicing for this length of time not only prevents your condition from worsening, but also builds up a great deal of Qi for the future.

If you can't commit to that much time, the next best thing is to practice twenty minutes a day, which is what the majority of people do. Either way, make the practice a part of your daily life, just as you would a shower. Doing Qigong once a day for twenty minutes gives you real prevention.

If you have a busy schedule, I always tell people to do the exercises as soon as they wake up or before going to bed. If you have a choice, it's best to do them in the evening rather than the morning. Did you know that if you practice for a quality twenty minutes at bedtime, the benefit is better than two to three hours of sleep?

Some people split the twenty minutes in half. You can do all ten movements, or just five—it doesn't matter which five. But *always* complete your practice by doing #10, *The Dragon Stands Between Heaven and Earth*. Remember, this is the exercise that brings you into a state of harmony and balance.

Remember, you can also do any of the movements alone. For example, you can do the kicks or the twists while waiting for a bus or subway, on line at the bank, or at your cafeteria at work. You can do the breathing exercise while watching television or do the toe dance at the beach. The only thing I ask is to be sure to practice each individual exercise for at least four to five minutes to get the maximum benefit out of your time and commitment.

If you don't have time during the week to do Qigong, then make the time over the weekend. That's still two or three days, which, although not the best, is better than nothing. A weekend practice will still give you a good tune-up. You also might want to eat more lightly—maybe just fruits or vegetables (both on and off the Recommended List)—on the weekend to give your stomach and internal organs a gentle cleaning.

If you don't do Qigong at all, then watch your diet and eat well. Another thing you can do for yourself is to take a break during the busiest hours of your day. For example, try stopping three or four times during the day for just two minutes each. One suggestion I tell people is to sit and close your eyes for 120 seconds before you start the engine in your car, or while you're commuting on the train or on the bus or as a passenger in a car. Take another two minutes while you're at your desk or on a break. If you practice this simple healing routine four times a day, that's eight minutes you've "stolen" back for yourself. If you can do it ten times a day, that's twenty minutes. You see, even two minutes can make a big difference in your life.

If you can't or don't do any of the above, then I'm sorry to say that you are not ready to heal or to change your life for the better. It is highly unlikely that you will find a unique program like this that cares so much about your whole self—your body, mind, spirit and emotions. It is highly unlikely you will encounter such wonderful healing knowledge that is based on an ancient medical system in continuous use for more than five thousand years. But I always tell my students and participants that you must leave a space for people to change. If you're one of the people with excess weight who is just not ready, I'll leave a space for you and wait for you to return to The Dragon's Way. I promise, you can be successful with The Dragon's Way. You can change; the power is literally in your hands.

CLOSING THOUGHTS

I hope this has been a good six weeks for you. One way to think about this experience is to imagine that you have created a magnificent garden. You have planted the seeds and have been diligently watering them. Some of the seeds may only have become little sprouts, barely pushing up through the ground. Other seeds have become young plants in just six weeks. And still other seeds have not yet sprouted and are quietly germinating below the surface, taking in the nourishment you are giving them. Whatever state your garden is in, you have to continue to take care of it—watering it, making certain that it gets enough sunlight, feeding the plants properly, and being sure that it doesn't become overgrown with weeds. If you take the time and cultivate it with love, your garden will become lush and healthy. But it is up to you to take care of your creation. In other words, it is up to you to take care of your life.

As you have now discovered, the world of TCM is an endless source of ancient wisdom that can help in very simple and practical ways. Its ancient teachings have been time-tested by millions and millions of people. The door to this practice is now finally open to people of the West. I am honored to be able to provide you with a special key through The Dragon's Way.

If you allow it, these ancient secrets of energy healing can help you change your life.

The Dragon's Way is now your way.

· ·

SOME FINAL TCM TIPS

USE YOUR INTUITION

Listen to your body, not your mind, when selecting foods and determining what you eat. Try closing your eyes for an instant in the supermarket. Your first idea (the first food that comes to mind) is what your body needs. Knowing what your body wants is a gift. The Dragon's Way helps the body recall this ability.

EAT "SOFTLY"

Try not to eat while you're having a meeting. Don't converse or talk on the phone while you're eating: talking and eating at the same time reverses the Qi or energy relationship between the stomach and the lung.

CHEW!

Chew your food well—it makes the digestive process easier for the body as a whole.

SEVENTY PERCENT IS BEST!

Eat until 70 percent full—this also makes the digestive process easier. Don't eat as if your mouth belongs to you and your stomach belongs to someone else!

YOUR MOTHER WAS RIGHT!

Heaviest food should be eaten earlier in the day. Eat a quality breakfast (e.g., toasted walnuts and fruit). Don't eat late at night. By the way, the most valuable part of the walnut is the "screen" between the two halves. It has a lot of energy that can be used to strengthen your kidney function. Some people like to make a tea of them.

COOKED, NOT RAW
Eat foods cooked, not raw. Save your Qi for healing.

HOW TO WET YOUR WHISTLE
Never drink iced fluids, especially when thirsty or after strenuous exercise.

JUICING WATERMELON AND OTHER COLD FACTS
Sometimes to gain the healing benefit of a particular food, it is necessary to eat it in large quantities. Juicing offers one way to eat more of the whole fruit of the watermelon. If you don't have a juicer, you can use a blender. Just cut up the watermelon into smaller pieces that the blender can handle. Everything in the watermelon has a healing benefit. Include the seeds, white and green (skin) part of the melon, as well as the red fruit. The seeds are a digestive aid. The roots and leaves of the plant can be used to make healthful soup.

TAKE A PASS WHEN THEY PASS FRIED AND BARBECUED FOODS
These foods cause excess internal heat. This is heat you definitely don't need or want. Continually experiencing internal heat is a health hazard which, at the very least, causes skin problems. So do yourself a favor—take a pass on these kinds of foods.

TAKING OFF THE CHILL
If your feet are cold in the winter, a quick way to bring warmth is by soaking them in a small tub of warm water. To warm cold hands and feet, put tangerine rind, black pepper, and ginger in boiling water for about ten minutes. Let the mixture cool down a bit so it's comfortable on your skin, then use the heated liquid as a wash for the cold parts of your body, or someone else's for that matter.

PMS? HERE'S SOME RELIEF

To reduce PMS symptoms, cover your legs in the winter and in the wind with something heavy, such as woolen pants or a long skirt. Pantyhose is not enough protection for the many meridians of your leg. For a PMS tea, place sliced ginger, scallion, orange peel, rose petals, rosemary, and cinnamon in a pot of water and bring to a boil. Reduce heat and let it steep for a few minutes. Drink the liquid hot twice a day when symptoms are present.

A FEW ANCIENT HEALING TIPS

If you bruise yourself or incur a sports injury, do not use ice—use heat on the bruise or rub some Tiger Balm or herbal wine on it. You can find herbal wines in most Chinese grocery stores, and a number of martial arts supply companies sell Tiger Balm. Another easy way to apply heat is to use Tabasco sauce. For centuries, TCM has successfully practiced the use of heat on sports injuries. While ice may numb the pain in the present, its cold essence can travel deep into your bones and cause you great arthritic pain later. Many athletes, famous and not so famous, have been forced to give up their game or retire because of serious arthritis. You can prevent this problem by switching to the use of heat now.

Have a minor burn? Apply the white of an egg—beaten or plain. What to do about a stomachache? Soak garlic in vinegar and sugar for a few months. Keep this mixture in a ceramic or glass jar with a closed top that you can store either in the refrigerator or on a shelf, then eat a clove when your stomach is bothering you.

ONE LAST TCM WORD OF ADVICE

Smile from your heart!

PART III
THE DRAGON'S FEAST
AND
MOST FREQUENTLY
ASKED QUESTIONS

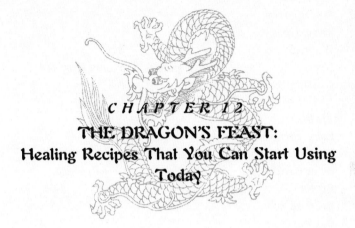

CHAPTER 12
THE DRAGON'S FEAST:
Healing Recipes That You Can Start Using Today

*O*NCE again, here is the list of recommended foods for The Dragon's Way. Following that is The Dragon's Feast, a compilation of delicious, inventive recipes using the healing foods in our program in tasty combinations. You may want to add your own recipes too.

FOODS FOR HEALING THE ROOT CAUSE OF EXCESS WEIGHT AND INCREASING QI

Fruits
 Kiwis
 Mangos
 Oranges
 Papaya
 Pears
 Persimmons
 Red apples (Gala, Macintosh, Washington State)
 Red grapefruit
 Red grapes

Strawberries
Tangerines
Watermelon
Note: There is a healing purpose to choosing red fruits, which is explained earlier.

Vegetables

Baby corn
Bamboo shoots
Bean curd
Broccoli
Broccoli rabe
Carrots
Cauliflower
Celery
Chicory
Eggplant
Fennel
Green peppers
Lotus
Mushrooms
Parsley
Plum tomatoes
Scallions
Seaweed (all kinds)
Water chestnuts
Yellow squash
Zucchini

Nuts/Spices/Oils

Black and white pepper
Black and white sesame seeds
Cashews
Chestnuts
Chili pepper

Cinnamon
Cloves
Garlic
Ginger
Lotus seed
Mint
Olive oil
Pine nuts
Safflower oil
Salt
Sesame oil
Soy sauce
Walnuts
Walnut oil

Others

Bee pollen
Coffee
Egg whites, cooked
Honey
Pasta (any kind)
Rice (any kind)
Tea (preferably Chinese herbal tea)

RECOMMENDED MEALS

Suggested Breakfast

Toasted walnuts (ten halves) and one of the following:

(a) one glass of watermelon juice (including some of the white and green parts of the rind). You can make watermelon juice with a juicer or a blender. For a blender, you will need to cut up the rind into smaller parts.

(b) apple juice

(c) orange juice

(d) one piece of recommended fruit

Lunch

Two pieces of recommended fruit. For red grapes and strawberries, eat a cup of fruit or more if you feel hungry. In the beginning, before you build up your Qi reserves with *Wu Ming* Meridian Therapy, you may need a little extra food in the morning. You can add more roasted walnuts and more fruit if you like.

Dinner

Two or three portions of recommended vegetables. Try to eat a variety of recommended vegetables at each meal. See if you can prepare three different-colored vegetables. Each color belongs to and can help heal a specific organ, according to The Five Element Theory. For example, baby corn is yellow and is good for your stomach and spleen; celery is green and is good for your liver; fennel is white and is good for your lung and kidney. These vegetables may be steamed, sautéed, stir-fried, braised, roasted, grilled, or prepared as soup. Do not fry, deep fry, or barbecue. Eat more if you feel hungry. You can also add a half-cup of any kind of rice or pasta.

THE DRAGON'S FEAST: HEALING RECIPES THAT YOU CAN BEGIN USING TODAY

Toasted Walnuts

DIRECTIONS:

Spread the walnuts in a single layer on a baking sheet. Put them in an oven that has been preheated to 325° and bake for about 15–20 minutes.

Or, put the walnuts in a frying pan or wok on the stove. No additional oil is necessary; the walnuts will have enough natural oil for cooking. Stirring constantly, sauté on medium heat for about 10 minutes. Store in a covered container.

Note: Unless specified, you may use any of the recommended oils for any of the following recipes.

Steamed Garlic Broccoli

INGREDIENTS:
> 2 cups water
> 3 sliced garlic cloves
> 1/8 teaspoon salt
> 1/4 cup white grape juice (optional)
> 3–4 cups broccoli florets

DIRECTIONS:
1. Place the water, garlic, and salt in a large pot and bring to a boil.
2. Lower the heat to a simmer, add the white grape juice.
3. Add the broccoli florets and toss them well in the liquid.
4. Cover and steam a few minutes until the broccoli is bright green and slightly tender.

Makes 3–4 cups.

Eggplant with Soy Sauce

INGREDIENTS:
> 1 teaspoon minced ginger
> 2 garlic cloves, minced
> 2 tablespoons soy sauce
> 2 tablespoons lemon juice
> 2 tablespoons honey or sugar
> 1 teaspoon chili powder
> 2 tablespoons walnut oil
> 3 cups water
> 1 pound eggplant, peeled (if using the small Chinese eggplant, do not peel)
> 1 teaspoon sesame oil

DIRECTIONS:

1. Cut eggplant into ½-inch by ½-inch by 2-inch strips.
2. Combine ginger and garlic in a bowl and set aside.
3. Mix soy sauce, vinegar, honey/sugar, and chili powder.
4. In a preheated wok or large heavy skillet, add walnut oil and heat until the oil is very hot.
5. Add the ginger and garlic—stir-fry for 5 seconds.
6. Add eggplant into wok and sauté.
7. Add the soy sauce mixture and bring to a boil.
8. Add 2 cups water. Cover wok and bring to a boil. Simmer for 10–15 minutes.
9. Stir in sesame oil and serve.

Zesty Zucchini Stir-Fry

INGREDIENTS:

4 tablespoons oil
¼ teaspoon salt (or less to taste)
1 large zucchini, quartered and sliced into thin, bite-sized pieces (about 4 cups)
4 strawberries, sliced
1 teaspoon soy sauce
¼ teaspoon sugar

DIRECTIONS:

1. Heat wok or large heavy skillet until very hot.
2. Add and heat oil.
3. Add salt.
4. Immediately add zucchini and strawberries.
5. Add soy sauce and sugar; stir well.
6. Cover and cook for 3–5 minutes; be careful not to overcook.

Makes about 3 cups.

Slightly Spicy Garden Casserole

INGREDIENTS:

15 scallions, cut into 4-inch pieces
4 tablespoons walnut oil
2 medium zucchinis, sliced in ¹/₂-inch circles (about 4 cups)
1 medium eggplant, sliced in ¹/₂-inch circles (about 5 cups)
6 stalks celery, coarsely diced
1 large green pepper, sliced into strips
1 cup parsley, chopped
3 cloves garlic, chopped very fine
4 large tomatoes, sliced in ¹/₂-inch circles
Salt, pepper, and ground chili pepper to taste

DIRECTIONS:

1. Lightly sauté the scallions in 3 tablespoons oil in a heavy casserole until lightly tender; remove and set aside.
2. Alternate layers of zucchini and eggplant, sprinkling each layer with a very small amount of salt, pepper, and ground chili pepper and some of the scallions.
3. Make a layer of celery and then green pepper. Sprinkle this layer with ¹/₈ teaspoon ground chili pepper.
4. Make a layer of the parsley and garlic and drizzle the remaining tablespoon of oil over it.
5. Layer the tomatoes over the top and sprinkle salt, pepper, and ground chili pepper over them. Cover.
6. Bring to a boil and simmer slowly for about 30 minutes or until the vegetables are tender.

Makes about 8 servings.

Zucchini with Walnuts

INGREDIENTS:

¹/₂ cup walnuts, coarsely chopped
1 tablespoon walnut oil

6–8 small zucchinis (about 1 pound)
Salt and freshly ground black pepper

DIRECTIONS:

1. Toast walnuts in a fry pan or a wok over medium heat until lightly browned (about 10 minutes). Remove from the heat and set aside.
2. Slice the zucchinis into ³/₄-inch pieces.
3. Heat wok or frying pan.
4. Add oil and heat.
5. Add the zucchini and stir-fry until it begins to soften.
6. Toss the walnuts in with the zucchini and add salt and pepper to taste.
7. Continue cooking until the zucchini is done.

Masterful Mushroom Sauté

INGREDIENTS:

2 tablespoons oil
2 scallions (cut into 1-inch pieces, separate the white and green parts)
2 slices fresh ginger
¹/₂ teaspoon sugar
1 pound of your favorite mushrooms, sliced
1 teaspoon soy sauce or ¹/₃ teaspoon salt
1–2 tablespoons oyster sauce
1 teaspoon cornstarch, dissolved in ¹/₄ cup cold water
1 tablespoon white grape juice
A few drops sesame oil

DIRECTIONS:

1. Heat wok or heavy skillet until very hot.
2. Add walnut oil.
3. Add white part of scallions and ginger.
4. When the scallions and ginger begin to cook (become aromatic), add the sugar and mushrooms.

5. Stir occasionally until the mushrooms are reduced by a third.
6. Stir in the soy sauce and the oyster sauce.
7. Add the green part of the scallions.
8. Remove some of the liquid from the pan and mix it into the dissolved cornstarch, then return this mixture to the pan.
9. Cook a few minutes until the sauce is thickened.
10. Add white grape juice and sesame oil.

Mexicali Mushrooms

Chunky Salsa

INGREDIENTS:

3 tablespoons walnut oil
3 cups scallions (whites and greens), finely chopped
3 cups green peppers, coarsely diced
1 teaspoon black pepper
1 teaspoon salt
2 pounds diced tomatoes, preferably peeled (plum tomatoes are best)
1/2 cup lemon juice
Salt and pepper

DIRECTIONS:

1. In a preheated wok or large heavy skillet, heat the oil and add the scallions, green pepper, pepper, and salt.
2. Cook until the scallions are slightly wilted; stir occasionally.
3. Purée half the tomatoes in a blender.
4. Add the puréed tomatoes and the diced tomatoes to the scallions and peppers in the wok and simmer on low heat for 10 minutes.

5. Stir in the lemon juice and heat for an additional few minutes.

Makes about 6–7 cups of salsa.

Mushrooms

INGREDIENTS:
>*1/4 cup water*
>*1 1/2 pounds mushrooms, quartered*
>*4 stalks celery, sliced*
>*Salt and pepper to taste*

DIRECTIONS:
1. In a preheated wok or large heavy skillet, combine all ingredients.
2. Cover and simmer on medium heat until the mushrooms are cooked to the tenderness you prefer, stirring occasionally.
3. Drain the excess liquid.
4. Place the mushrooms on a platter and cover with some of the salsa.

Mushroom Soup

INGREDIENTS:
>*3 pounds mushrooms (any kind you like)*
>*1 1/2 quarts water*
>*1 bunch parsley, about 3 cups*
>*2 cloves garlic*
>*1 teaspoon salt*
>*1/4 teaspoon pepper*
>*4 tablespoons oil*
>*2 large bunches scallions, cut into 1-inch pieces, greens only*
>*6 stalks celery, sliced thin*
>*1/4 cup soy sauce*

DIRECTIONS:

1. Wash the mushrooms. Dice half of them and thinly slice the other half. Use all the stems, because they will be puréed.
2. In a saucepan, bring 1 quart of water to a boil and add the diced mushrooms.
3. Reduce the heat, cover, and simmer until they are tender.
4. Wash the parsley and chop coarsely, removing the bottom stems; set aside.
5. In a blender, purée the cooked mushrooms with the parsley, garlic, salt, and pepper in small batches and set aside.
6. In a soup pot, heat the oil, add the scallions, celery, and soy sauce. Cook until the celery is slightly tender.
7. Toss in the sliced mushrooms, cover and cook for 5 minutes on medium heat.
8. Add the remaining 2 cups of water, stir, and bring to a boil.
9. Add the purée, reduce heat, and simmer for about 5 minutes.

Makes about 12 cups of soup.

Cauliflower Stew

INGREDIENTS:

2 cups water
1 large head cauliflower, cored and quartered
2 tablespoons walnut, sesame, or safflower oil
3 cloves garlic, crushed
4 stalks celery, thinly sliced
1 cup fennel root, slivered
1/2 green pepper, chopped
7 large plum tomatoes, quartered and sliced
1 large bunch scallions (8–10); chop green and white parts coarsely

Salt and pepper to taste
Several sprigs parsley, chopped

DIRECTIONS:

1. Bring the water to boil in a large pot and add the cauliflower.
2. Cover and steam until the cauliflower is very tender (about 5 minutes). Set aside.
3. Heat the oil in a preheated wok or large, heavy skillet.
4. Add the garlic and celery and cook until the celery begins to turn translucent.
5. Add the fennel and green pepper. Stir occasionally and cook until the green pepper turns a bright shade of green.
6. Add the plum tomatoes and scallions and toss all the vegetables together.
7. While the vegetables are cooking, mash the cauliflower slightly and then return it to the wok or skillet.
8. Season with salt and pepper to taste.
9. Serve with chopped parsley on top.

Serving suggestion: Sprinkle a little cinnamon on top just before serving, especially if you have used sesame oil.

Tomato Zucchini Soup

INGREDIENTS:

4 tablespoons oil
1/2 teaspoon salt
1–2 cloves garlic, crushed
1 stalk celery, diced
2 scallions (separate white and green parts), diced
2–3 1/8-inch thick slices of fresh ginger
2 small or 1 medium zucchini
5 medium-to-large plum tomatoes, diced
1/8 teaspoon sugar
1/2 cup water
1/4 cup white grape juice

DIRECTIONS:

1. In a preheated wok or large, heavy skillet, heat half of the oil until very hot.
2. Add salt, garlic, celery, whites of scallion, and ginger.
3. Sauté until celery begins to turn translucent.
4. Add zucchini and stir-fry until tender.
5. Remove ingredients from wok and set aside.
6. Reheat wok and add oil; continue to heat until the oil is very hot.
7. Add diced tomatoes and sugar and cook until the juice is released (about 5 minutes).
8. Mix the zucchini in with the tomatoes and cook another 5 minutes.
9. Add the water, white grape juice, and green scallions. Cook another 5 minutes. Serve hot.

When it is puréed, this soup also makes an excellent sauce for use over other vegetables.

Mushrooms Stuffed with Roasted Eggplant

INGREDIENTS:

1 large eggplant
1 tablespoon sesame oil
2 cups plum tomatoes, finely diced and quartered
¼ teaspoon salt and pepper to taste
1 clove garlic, finely chopped
2 tablespoons parsley, chopped
1 tablespoon lemon juice
24 large mushrooms with the stems removed

DIRECTIONS:

1. Place the eggplant in a baking dish that has 1 inch of water in it and bake at 350° for about 30 minutes.
2. Remove it when it is very soft to the touch and let it cool.

3. When it is cool, peel it and remove the seeds.
4. Mash the remainder of the eggplant until fairly smooth (the eggplant should be cooked till it is almost custard-like in texture).
5. Heat a wok or heavy skillet and add the sesame oil.
6. Add tomatoes, salt, pepper, garlic, and parsley and stir-fry lightly.
7. Remove from heat and mix into the eggplant.
8. Add lemon juice and stir.
9. Lightly steam the mushroom caps till tender.
10. Fill the caps with the eggplant.
11. Heat in a preheated 350° oven for a few minutes.

Serve warm.

Stuffed Peppers 1

INGREDIENTS:
>4 *small green bell peppers, halved and seeded*
>6 *tablespoons safflower or walnut oil*
>1 *small eggplant, peeled and chopped in 2-inch pieces*
>2 *cups of your favorite mushrooms*
>1 *cup plum tomatoes, diced*
>5 *scallions, chopped in 1/2-inch pieces*
>20 *toasted walnuts, chopped*
>1/2 *cup parsley leaves, chopped*
>1 *teaspoon salt*
>1/2 *teaspoon pepper*

DIRECTIONS:
1. Heat a wok or heavy skillet and add 4 tablespoons oil.
2. Add eggplant and mushrooms, stir-fry for 4–5 minutes.
3. Transfer ingredients to a large bowl.
4. Mix the tomatoes, scallions, parsley, walnuts, and salt and pepper into the eggplant and mushrooms.
5. Sprinkle a teaspoon of oil into each of the pepper halves.

6. Fill each pepper half with the vegetable mixture.
7. Place in a baking dish and cover with tin foil.
8. Bake for 30 minutes at 325°.

Stuffed Peppers II

INGREDIENTS:

4 large green peppers
1 head chicory
1 cup bamboo shoots, finely chopped
1 tablespoon soy sauce
½ teaspoon black pepper
2 cups apple juice

DIRECTIONS:

1. Cut off the tops of the peppers and set aside.
2. Remove the seeds and rinse the peppers out without breaking them.
3. Carefully wash the chicory and shred finely.
4. Mix the chicory, bamboo shoots, soy sauce, black pepper, and 1 cup of apple juice together and stuff into the peppers.
5. Place the tops back on the peppers and fasten them with toothpicks.
6. Place upright in a nonstick baking dish with the rest of the apple juice on the bottom of the pan.
7. Bake for 30 minutes at 325°.

Grilled Vegetables

INGREDIENTS:

Zucchini
Plum tomatoes, cut in half
Celery, cut in 2-inch pieces
Mushrooms
Green peppers, cut in strips

DIRECTIONS:

1. On separate skewers, place large chunks of zucchini, plum tomato halves, 2-inch pieces of celery, mushrooms, and strips of green pepper on skewers. Brush each skewer with oil.
2. Zucchini will grill in about 15 minutes; mushrooms, 10 minutes; tomatoes, 5 minutes; celery, 8 minutes; green pepper strips, 5 minutes.

Grilling tips: Mushrooms will grill in about 5 minutes and retain their moisture if preboiled for a few minutes before grilling.

Baked Breakfast Apples

INGREDIENTS:

> 1 large red apple per person
> 1 tablespoon toasted walnuts, chopped
> 1/4 teaspoon cinnamon
> 1/4 teaspoon honey

DIRECTIONS:

1. Preheat oven to 400°.
2. Wash and core apple; do not remove skin.
3. Fill the core of the apple with the walnuts, cinnamon, and honey.
4. Place the apple(s) in a baking dish with about 1/4 cup of water in the bottom of the dish.
5. Bake at 400° for approximately 45 minutes or until the apple is soft.

Warm Apple Soup

INGREDIENTS:

> 3 cups water
> 2 peeled and cored large red apples, cut into small sticks
> 2 inches ginger, peeled and diced finely

1 tablespoon honey
Zest of 1 orange peel

DIRECTIONS:
1. Place the water in a saucepan and bring to a boil.
2. Add the apples and ginger and reduce the heat to a simmer.
3. Simmer slowly until the apples are very soft, about 10 minutes; liquid should have reduced by one-third.
4. Add honey, stir.
5. Sprinkle the orange zest over the soup before serving.

Makes 3 cups.
Note: This is great for breakfast!

Apple Pear Compote

INGREDIENTS:
3 red apples
3 ripe pears
1 cup water
1/2 teaspoon cinnamon
10 toasted walnuts, chopped coarsely for garnish

DIRECTIONS:
1. Peel and core pears and apples and cut into 1/2-inch slices.
2. Place fruit into a 3-quart pot, add water and cinnamon.
3. Cover and cook over medium heat for approximately 20 minutes or until fruit is soft.
4. Remove from heat and serve warm with chopped toasted walnuts on top.

Gingered Orange/Mango

INGREDIENTS:
2 medium mangos
2 large juice oranges

1 teaspoon cornstarch
3/4 teaspoon fresh ginger root, grated
1/8 teaspoon salt

DIRECTIONS:

1. Peel and cut mangos off the pit into large chunks and set aside.
2. In a small bowl, mix the juice from the two oranges (which should equal about 1/2 cup) and the cornstarch.
3. Add to this mixture the ginger with some of the orange pulp and the salt.
4. Pour it into a heated wok or heavy skillet and cook and stir over medium heat until it begins to thicken and bubbles.
5. Add the mango chunks and cook, stirring for another minute and coating the mango pieces with the orange ginger sauce.

Serve warm.

Strawberry Sauce

INGREDIENTS:

2 cups fresh strawberries
1/4 cup honey or sugar, adjust to tartness of fruit
1 tablespoon lemon juice
1/2 teaspoon cinnamon
1 teaspoon cornstarch
2 tablespoons water

DIRECTIONS:

1. Clean berries well and quarter them.
2. Place them in a saucepan with the honey and lemon juice.
3. Cover and cook for 10 minutes, stirring occasionally.
4. Stir in the cinnamon.

5. Purée mixture in a blender and return them to the saucepan.
6. Mix the cornstarch and water together until smooth and add slowly to the hot fruit.
7. Cook mixture over low heat, stirring constantly until it is clear and thickened.

Makes approximately 1 cup of sauce.

Traditional Cooked Pears

INGREDIENTS:
6 chopped pears, any variety
¹/₃ cup rock sugar candy
¹/₄ cup water

DIRECTIONS:
1. Place all the ingredients in a 2-quart double boiler.
2. Cook on low heat for about 40 minutes.
3. Eat a few tablespoons a day.

Note: This recipe is particularly good for helping those with the flu caused by heat. How do you know if you have this kind of flu? Symptoms are a sore throat and fever.

Broccoli Rabe with Tomato Sauce

Sauce:

INGREDIENTS:
3 tablespoons oil
2 cloves garlic, crushed
¹/₂ stalk celery, chopped finely
1 bunch (about 10) young scallions, chopped in ¹/₄-inch pieces; use the white and green parts
¹/₂ green pepper, chopped finely
4 mushrooms, chopped finely
³/₄ cup fresh parsley, chopped

¹/₄ teaspoon black pepper
1 teaspoon salt
1 teaspoon sugar
1 pound plum tomatoes, diced

DIRECTIONS:

1. Add oil to a heated wok or large heavy skillet.
2. Add the garlic and celery and cook until the celery begins to become translucent.
3. Add the scallions and green pepper and cook until the scallions are fully wilted.
4. Add the rest of the ingredients, reserving 2 teaspoons of the parsley for garnish.
5. Cover and simmer gently for about 1 hour, stirring occasionally.
6. Remove the lid and continue cooking until the sauce thickens a little.

Broccoli Rabe:

INGREDIENTS:

1 quart boiling, lightly salted water
1 tablespoon oil
1 bunch broccoli rabe, about ¹/₂ pound
1 large clove garlic, minced

DIRECTIONS:

1. Thoroughly clean the broccoli rabe and trim the ends.
2. Place broccoli rabe in the pot of boiling, salted water for about 2 minutes.
3. Remove them from the pot and set aside.
4. In a heated wok or large heavy skillet add oil, and when the oil is very hot, add the broccoli rabe.
5. Lightly stir-fry and add the garlic in the last two minutes.
6. Place the broccoli rabe lengthwise on a platter and pour the tomato sauce across the center of the stalks. Sprinkle the 2 teaspoons of parsley over the sauce for color.

Cooked Watermelon Rind

INGREDIENTS:

 2 teaspoons safflower oil

 3–4 chopped scallions, separate the white and the green

 2 cups of the white part of the watermelon rind, cut into
  1-inch cubes

 1/2 teaspoon fresh ginger root, sliced

 1 teaspoon soy sauce

DIRECTIONS:

1. Heat wok or heavy skillet until very hot, then add oil.
2. Add the white part of the scallions and cook until tender.
3. Add melon cubes and ginger.
4. Stir-fry until the melon begins to sweat heavily.
5. Add soy sauce and green part of scallions.
6. Sitr-fry for another minute.

Walnuts and Black Sesame Seeds

INGREDIENTS:

 1/2 pound walnuts

 1/2 pound black sesame seeds

 3–4 ounces honey

DIRECTIONS:

1. Grind walnuts and black sesame seeds together in
   blender.
2. Cook in a double boiler or steam for 1 hour.
3. Thoroughly mix in honey.
4. After cooking, refrigerate.
5. Eat 2 tablespoons in the morning. (After the program,
   you can eat an additional 2 teaspoons in the evening
   as well.)

Ratatouille

INGREDIENTS:

1 medium eggplant
Large bowl with salted water
1 large green pepper
5 large plum tomatoes
3 small zucchinis
½ cup oil
10–12 young scallions
½ teaspoon ground black pepper
½ cup parsley, chopped
1 teaspoon honey

DIRECTIONS:

1. Cut the unpeeled eggplant lengthwise into ½-inch slices.
2. Place slices into the bowl with enough salted water to cover the eggplant and press the eggplant down with a plate, putting something heavy on top of the plate to keep the eggplant submerged. Let slices soak for about 20 minutes.
3. Cut the pepper into strips, chop the tomatoes into chunks, and slice the zucchinis lengthwise in ¼-inch strips.
4. Heat one-half the oil in a wok or large skillet.
5. Add the scallions, pepper, and zucchini, and cover. Cook for about 5 minutes.
6. Drain the eggplant and pat dry.
7. Mix the eggplant with the zucchini mixture.
8. Add the rest of the oil; cover and cook for 5 minutes.
9. Mix in the tomatoes, pepper, parsley, and honey.
10. Cook for another 5–15 minutes.

Confetti Eggplant

INGREDIENTS:

 2 tablespoons oil
 ½ cup cauliflower, chopped
 ½ cup broccoli florets
 1 medium eggplant, cut into small chunks
 ½ cup water
 ½ cup green pepper, diced
 1 teaspoon salt
 1 teaspoon chili pepper
 4 plum tomatoes, diced
 1 small can bamboo shoots
 2 scallions, cut into ½-inch pieces

DIRECTIONS:

1. Heat wok or large skillet and add oil.
2. Add cauliflower, broccoli, and sauté lightly; remove from wok.
3. Put the eggplant and water in the wok and cook until tender.
4. Mix in the green pepper, salt, chili pepper, and tomatoes. Cook until the tomatoes just begin to soften.
5. Return the cauliflower and broccoli to the wok along with the bamboo shoots and scallions.
6. Cook for about 5 minutes and serve.

Eggplant Soup or Eggplant Cleansing Drink

Eggplant has special healing properties that are particularly good for cleansing the liver and taking off weight. TCM practitioners also use eggplant to heal hepatitis. This recipe may be served hot as a soup, or at room temperature as a vegetable "cocktail." Drinking a cup a day can help speed weight reduction.

INGREDIENTS:

 5 cups peeled eggplant (makes about 1 cup of juice)
 5–7 scallions, white part only

2 large stalks celery

2 cloves garlic

2 large tomatoes (the celery and tomatoes make about 1 cup of juice)

1 teaspoon salt

1/2 teaspoon black pepper

Juice of 1 small lemon

1 tablespoon sugar (optional)

DIRECTIONS:

1. Juice all ingredients together.
2. Pour into saucepan and bring to a boil; reduce heat.
3. Add salt, pepper, and lemon juice (1 tablespoon sugar optional)
4. Simmer for 15 minutes.
5. Garnish with chopped parsley or watercress.

Note: After The Dragon's Way program, you can add cooked barley to this dish as a soup.

Stuffed Fennel

INGREDIENTS:

4 fennel bulbs

Large pot of boiling water, lightly salted

1/2 cup toasted pine nuts or crushed, toasted walnuts

1 cup parsley

1 teaspoon salt

1 teaspoon ground pepper

1/4 cup oil

DIRECTIONS:

1. Thoroughly wash the fennel bulbs in cold water, trim, and cut a core in the center.
2. Cook the fennel in boiling salted water for about 30 minutes or until tender; set aside to cool slightly.

3. Combine nuts, parsley, salt and pepper, and 1 teaspoon oil.
4. Stuff the nut mixture in the "core."
5. Place the fennel standing up in a baking dish and drizzle the remaining oil over them.
6. Bake at 325° for about 20 minutes or until they begin to brown slightly.

Mushrooms and Fennel

INGREDIENTS:

3 tablespoons oil (walnut oil is particularly good in this recipe)
7 scallions (about 1 cup), cut in 1-inch pieces
1 cup fennel bulb, chopped
2 stalks celery, sliced thinly
1/2 cup parsley leaves, chopped
2 pounds mushrooms, sliced
4 tablespoons fennel leaves, chopped
2 tablespoons soy sauce
1/2 teaspoon black pepper

DIRECTIONS:

1. Heat wok or large heavy skillet and add oil.
2. Add the scallions, fennel, and celery. Cover and cook until tender. Stir occasionally.
3. Toss in the parsley and mushrooms and cook on high heat for about 5 minutes until the mushrooms are tender, stirring occasionally.
4. Stir in the fennel leaves, soy sauce, and black pepper and cook for 2–3 more minutes.

Makes 4–6 cups.

Mushroom Sauce

INGREDIENTS:

    $\frac{1}{4}$ cup oil
    10 scallions, finely diced
    $\frac{1}{2}$ cup celery, diced
    1 pound mushrooms, finely diced
    1 cup plum tomatoes, chopped
    2 teaspoons salt
    1 teaspoon ground pepper
    1 teaspoon cornstarch
    $\frac{1}{4}$ cup apple juice

DIRECTIONS:

1. In a heated wok or heavy skillet, heat oil.
2. Add the diced scallions and celery and cook until the celery is translucent.
3. Mix in the mushrooms and cook until they are reduced by half.
4. Mix in the tomatoes, salt and pepper, and cook for about 15 minutes, stirring occasionally.
5. Mix the cornstarch into the apple juice until smooth and then slowly add to the mushroom mixture.
6. Cook until the sauce thickens slightly.

This sauce can also be used with stuffed zucchini, eggplant, or tomatoes.

Mushrooms, Bamboo Shoots, and Tomatoes

INGREDIENTS:

    2 tablespoons oil
    1 pound mushrooms
    4 plum tomatoes
    1 cup bamboo shoots
    $\frac{1}{4}$ cup soy sauce

¹/₄ teaspoon black pepper
    ¹/₂ cup lemon juice
    ¹/₂ cup sugar

DIRECTIONS:

1. Wash and quarter your favorite mushrooms.
2. In a preheated wok or large heavy skillet, heat oil and add the mushrooms.
3. Sauté on medium heat until tender.
4. Cut the tomatoes into quarters and then in half horizontally so that you have 8 "chunks" for each tomato; turn the heat up to high.
5. Mix the bamboo shoots and tomatoes into the mushrooms.
6. Mix the soy sauce, pepper, lemon juice, and sugar together and pour over the vegetables. Stir lightly, coating the vegetables with the liquid.
7. Adjust seasoning to taste and serve.

Makes approximately 4 to 6 cups.

Braised Chicory

INGREDIENTS:

    1 pound chicory
    3 tablespoons oil
    ¹/₂ cup scallions, finely diced
    1 cup bamboo shoots, finely chopped
    ¹/₄ cup parsley, finely cut
    ³/₄ cup apple juice
    ¹/₂ teaspoon salt
    ¹/₄ teaspoon pepper
    2 tablespoons sugar

DIRECTIONS:

1. Carefully wash the chicory to remove the grit that tends to get caught in its curly leaves and base.

2. Place it in a pan of boiling water for 1 minute, remove and put immediately into a bowl of cold water.
3. Dry the chicory well.
4. Place the scallion, bamboo shoots, and parsley in the bottom of a well-oiled baking dish.
5. Lay the chicory over the vegetables.
6. Add the oil, salt, pepper, and sugar to the apple juice and pour it over the chicory.
7. Cover with oiled wax paper or foil.
8. Cook at 325° for about 1 hour.
9. Remove the chicory and place on a serving plate.
10. Place the liquid and vegetables from the baking dish into a saucepan and reduce by half.
11. Pour over the chicory and serve.

Cooked Salad

INGREDIENTS:

> 3 cups boiling water
> Your favorite vegetable salad

DIRECTIONS:

1. Put your favorite salad in a pot of boiling water for 1–2 minutes to blanch and eliminate its cold essence.
2. Strain the salad and place on a platter.

Dressing:

INGREDIENTS:

> 2 tablespoons oil
> 1 clove garlic, minced
> 1 teaspoon salt
> 1/8 teaspoon pepper
> 1 teaspoon soy sauce
> 1 teaspoon ginger, grated

DIRECTIONS:

1. Put the oil and garlic in a heated wok or skillet.
2. Cook the garlic until it is almost burned.
3. Add the salt, pepper, soy sauce, and ginger.

Apples and Chicory

INGREDIENTS:

1 pound of chicory (about 1 large head), shredded
½ cup apple juice
¼ cup lemon juice
½ teaspoon salt
2 tablespoons sugar
1 tablespoon oil
2 large apples (about 4 cups), peeled, cored, and diced

DIRECTIONS:

1. Wash the chicory very carefully to remove all the grit that collects on its curly leaves. When shredding, do not use the white parts at the base of the head.
2. Mix together the apple juice, lemon juice, salt, and sugar.
3. In a preheated wok or large heavy skillet, heat the oil and add the apples, using high heat.
4. Stir occasionally and sauté the apples until they begin to soften and are reduced by about one-half.
5. Pour the juice mixture over it and toss all the ingredients together well.
6. Simmer until the chicory is cooked (about 1–2 minutes), stirring occasionally.
7. Drain off the liquid and serve immediately.

Lemon Broccoli

INGREDIENTS:

2 bunches broccoli, trimmed but left in spears
2 cups water

¹/₄ cup soy sauce
¹/₂ cup lemon juice
¹/₄ teaspoon black pepper
1 bunch broccoli

DIRECTIONS:

1. Mix the water, soy sauce, lemon juice and pepper together and pour into a heated wok or heavy large skillet and bring to a boil.
2. Place the broccoli spears in the wok and simmer until tender.

Baked Cauliflower

INGREDIENTS:

1 medium head cauliflower, chopped
3 cups celery, diced
1 cup boiling, slightly salted water
¹/₂ cup green pepper, chopped
¹/₄ cup scallions, chopped; use the white parts
1 teaspoon salt
¹/₂ teaspoon black pepper

DIRECTIONS:

1. Preheat oven to 350°.
2. In a saucepan, place the cauliflower and celery in the salted water and simmer for 5 minutes. Remove the cauliflower and celery from the pan and save the liquid.
3. Place the cauliflower and celery in a lightly oiled baking pan.
4. Add green pepper and scallions to ³/₄ cup of the liquid with the salt and pepper and pour over the top of the cauliflower and celery. Cover.
5. Bake about 30 minutes.

Cauliflower Chinese-Style

INGREDIENTS:

    5 tablespoons oil
    1/4 teaspoon salt
    2 scallions, white part only
    1 small cauliflower, chopped into bite-size pieces
    1/4 teaspoon sugar
    1/4 teaspoon water
    Splash of white grape juice

DIRECTIONS:

1. Heat oil in a preheated wok.
2. Add salt and scallions.
3. Immediately add cauliflower and stir-fry for 2 minutes.
4. Add sugar.
5. Stir in water.
6. Cover and cook for a few minutes until it is aromatic.
7. Stirring quickly, add grape juice.

Nutty Celery

INGREDIENTS:

    2 tablespoons walnut oil
    4 cups celery stalks (8–10 large stalks), sliced
    1/4 teaspoon pepper
    1 small garlic clove, finely chopped
    2 tablespoons scallion greens, chopped
    1 cup toasted walnuts, chopped
    1 ripe persimmon, quartered and sliced (preferably the round persimmon that can be eaten hard rather than the acorn-shaped persimmon)
    1/2 cup apple juice

DIRECTIONS:

1. In a preheated wok or large skillet, place oil, celery, pepper, garlic, and scallions; mix.

2. Cover and cook over low heat until the celery is tender but still slightly crunchy. Stir occasionally.

3. When the celery is tender, place it on a medium serving dish and cover.

4. Put the toasted, chopped walnuts, sliced persimmon, and apple juice in the wok and heat thoroughly, about 2–3 minutes; liquid will be absorbed or evaporated.

5. Pour over the celery and serve immediately.

Makes 4–6 servings.

Tomato Sauce

INGREDIENTS:

> 2 tablespoons oil
> 1 garlic clove, crushed
> 1 cup scallions, finely chopped
> 1 teaspoon salt
> ½ teaspoon pepper
> 2 pounds plum tomatoes, chopped
> 1 teaspoon sugar
> 1 teaspoon parsley

DIRECTIONS:

1. Heat oil in a large skillet or wok.

2. Add garlic, scallions, salt and pepper, and sauté lightly.

3. Add tomatoes, sugar, and parsley.

4. Cover and simmer over low heat for 1 hour, stirring occasionally.

5. Remove lid and cook over low heat until the sauce thickens.

TCM Tea Remedy for Colds

INGREDIENTS:

> 3 cups water
> 2–3 inches fresh ginger root, sliced

4–5 scallions, white part only
Peel of 2 tangerines

DIRECTIONS:

1. Place all of the above ingredients into a pot of 3 cups of water.
2. Bring it to boil, reduce heat, and simmer for no more than 3–4 minutes.
3. Strain the ingredients and drink hot.

If you want to sweeten this tea, use brown sugar or honey.

AFTER THE DRAGON'S WAY PROGRAM

Here are a few recipes that help strengthen your Qi that you can add into your Eating for Healing plan after The Dragon's Way.

Breakfast

INGREDIENTS:

Dried white fungus (actually a flowery looking mushroom available in oriental markets; should be soaked overnight in 1 quart of water. About ¹/₂ of one piece should be sufficient.)
¹/₂ cup dried chestnuts, chopped
¹/₂ cup dried red dates
¹/₄ cup lily bulb (choose white ones, not yellow ones. The yellow ones can have a sour taste when cooked.)
¹/₄ cup pearl barley
¹/₂ cup dried lotus seed (soak overnight in water)
¹/₄ cup lyceum fruit (wolfberry—can be found in health food stores)
Rock candy sugar, coconut cream, or honey.

DIRECTIONS:

1. Mix all of the ingredients together in 1 quart of water, bring to boil.

2. Add sweetener after ingredients have cooked at least a half hour. The cereal is done when the barley is tender.

Makes 2–4 servings.

This recipe has a lot of nutrition and energy and is good to use after the program. It is a fun and optional recipe. You can easily leave out one or more of the ingredients and it will still provide nutritional benefits. Experiment with the combination that you like the best. You can cook this as a sweet dessert or for breakfast instead of your usual cereal.

Red Bean and Chinese Barley Soup

INGREDIENTS:
   8 ounces Chinese pearl barley
   4 ounces small red beans
   4 ounces lily bulb
   4 ounces dried lotus seed
   2 quarts water
   Dried tangerine peel
   Rock sugar candy or granulated sugar to taste (optional)

DIRECTIONS:
   Crock Pot Method:
   1. Place all ingredients in crock pot. Cook for several hours or until beans are well-cooked.

   Stovetop Method:
   1. Place all ingredients in a large pot and bring to a boil.
   2. Lower heat to medium and simmer for approximately 1 hour or until beans are well-cooked.

Three Seeds Soup

INGREDIENTS:

- 4 teaspoons sesame oil
- 5 garlic cloves, smashed
- 1 carrot, chopped
- 2 celery stalks, chopped
- 4 ounces Chinese white beans (shen bian dou)[1] (soaked overnight)
- 4 ounces Chinese small red beans (soaked overnight)
- 4 ounces dried white lotus seed (buy only the white ones—if they are yellow, they are old)
- 5–6 cups water
- Salt and pepper to taste
- Pinch of cornstarch
- 2–3 plum tomatoes, chopped

Optional additions: walnuts, water chestnuts, honey

DIRECTIONS:

1. In a preheated wok, add and heat the sesame oil.
2. Add garlic, carrot, celery, beans, lotus seeds, salt and pepper, and stir-fry slightly.
3. At this point, add the (optional) water chestnuts and walnuts, if desired.
4. Add water so that it covers the ingredients by 2 inches and bring to a boil.
5. Lower heat to medium and simmer for about 1 hour or until beans are soft. Add water as needed, stir occasionally.
6. Add a pinch of cornstarch and tomatoes.
7. For a sweet soup, add honey.

---

[1]The white and red beans are actually seeds that have a very healthful effect on the body.

Barley Soup

INGREDIENTS:

- ½ cup Chinese pearl barley
- 5 cups water
- 1 broccoli stalk with the tough outer skin cut off, or 1 stalk celery
- 1 medium green pepper, cored, seeded and chopped into bite-sized pieces
- 5–6 tomatoes, cut in small pieces
- ½ teaspoon vinegar
- ⅓ cup parsley, chopped
- 1 teaspoon salt
- ½ teaspoon black pepper
- 1 tablespoon walnut oil

DIRECTIONS:

1. Rinse barley.
2. Place the water in a 3- or 4-quart soup pot and bring to a boil.
3. Add the barley and reduce heat to medium; simmer for 30 minutes.
4. Heat wok and add oil.
5. When the oil is very hot, add broccoli or celery stalk, peppers and tomatoes, ½ teaspoon salt, and ¼ teaspoon pepper.
6. Sauté for 5–10 minutes until the juices are released.
7. Add the vegetables to the barley.
8. Add vinegar, parsley, and remaining salt and pepper.
9. Cook on low heat for another 30 minutes.
10. Adjust seasonings to taste.

Creamy Mushroom Barley Soup

INGREDIENTS:

- ¾ cups Chinese pearl barley
- 6 cups water

4 cups cauliflower, cut into small pieces
1 tablespoon walnut oil
1⅓ cups mushrooms, sliced
1⅓ cups celery, finely chopped
2 scallions, chopped
1¼ teaspoons salt
1 teaspoon black pepper

DIRECTIONS:

1. Rinse barley.
2. Place the water in a 3–4 quart soup pot and bring to a boil.
3. Add the barley and reduce heat to medium; cover and simmer for 30 minutes.
4. In a separate pot, steam cauliflower until tender.
5. Pureé cauliflower and set aside.
6. Heat wok and add oil.
7. When the oil is very hot, add mushrooms, celery, and scallions.
8. Sauté for 5–10 minutes until the juices are released.
9. Add the vegetables and cauliflower purée to the barley.
10. Season with salt and pepper.
11. Cook on low heat until soup thickens.
12. Adjust seasonings to your own taste.

Vegetable Purée Soup

INGREDIENTS:

3 tablespoons walnut oil
Salt and pepper
2 stalks celery, diced
2 scallions, diced
3–4 recommended vegetables of your choice cut into bite-size pieces
3 cups water
Pinch of cinnamon

DIRECTIONS:

1. In a preheated wok or large heavy skillet, add oil and heat until it is very hot.
2. Add salt and pepper, celery, and scallions, and sauté.
3. Add your chosen vegetables and stir.
4. Add water and bring to a boil; simmer until vegetables are soft.
5. Remove the vegetables from the broth and set the broth aside.
6. Purée vegetables and return them to the broth and stir well.
7. Reheat and add cinnamon.
8. Adjust seasonings to taste.

Our Favorite Shrimp Sauté

INGREDIENTS:

2 tablespoons cold water

1 teaspoon cornstarch

2 egg whites

24 deveined shrimp, sliced in half lengthwise

Walnut or other light oil

1 teaspoon salt

2 scallions, chopped

1/2 cup sugar

2 medium tomatoes, cut into small chunks

1 medium peach, cut into small chunks

1/4 cup wine (optional)

1 teaspoon sesame oil

5–10 toasted walnuts, crushed

DIRECTIONS:

1. Mix water and cornstarch together and stir into the egg whites.

2. Put the shrimp in the egg whites and coat them well; let them soak in the egg white mixture.
3. Heat wok, add the oil, and heat the oil very hot.
4. Add salt and scallions to walnut oil and sauté lightly.
5. Add sugar and stir.
6. Add tomato and peach; sauté until they just begin to release their juices.
7. Add shrimp and sauté until they have changed color.
8. Add wine and then sesame oil; stir lightly.
9. Turn onto serving dish and sprinkle with crushed walnuts.

Makes 4 servings.

Healing Bean Recipe for Strengthening the Digestive System

There are no exact amounts given in this recipe. This is an ancient dish adapted to address Western health needs. Using the basic proportions and ingredients, cook by intuition and taste for seasonings.

DIRECTIONS:

Soak 2 times as many small white beans to small red beans overnight. You can also add dry chestnuts and/or black beans in the same proportion of red beans to white beans. (For example, if you use ½ pound of dry white beans, use ¼ pound of dry small red beans, ¼ pound of dry black beans and/or ¼ pound of dry chestnuts.) Note: small red beans and small white beans must be used!

Put cold sesame (or other) oil in a preheated wok or large heavy skillet and heat until it just begins to smoke.

Add about 5 cloves of chopped garlic and a little salt.

Then add the beans and sauté until the beans are heated. Add a little more salt and ½ teaspoon of sugar.

Add a stalk of celery and a carrot, diced. Stir and cook until the mixture begins to sweat. Be careful not to burn the beans. Add enough water to cover 1 inch above the beans. Bring to a boil. Stir well. Reduce heat to low, cover and simmer for about 2 hours or until beans are tender. If water is reduced, add more water. When it is almost done, season it to taste. You can also add sliced tomatoes.

Keep this in your refrigerator. Eat a little when you are hungry or have it for lunch or breakfast every day. It is too heavy to eat for dinner. After three or four weeks, there should be a positive change in your digestion. It should be stronger and also, if you are retaining excess water, this healing recipe should help eliminate it. This recipe can also increase your Qi. It is particularly good for people who suffer from chronic fatigue syndrome or are in a weakened condition from an operation.

Chicken with Ginseng

INGREDIENTS:
> 1 small baby or spring chicken[1]
> 1 ounce American ginseng[2]
> 3 slices (about 2 inches) ginger root
> ½ cup red wine

DIRECTIONS:
1. Wash the chicken and cut it into 8 pieces.
2. Put all the ingredients into a crock pot.
3. Add boiling water to 1 inch above the chicken.
4. Simmer for several hours.

Eat once or twice a week.

---

[1]Note about choosing chicken: chickens are often "processed" and raised with hormonal supplements to force them to grow faster. Purchase natural, free-range, or unprocessed chickens.
[2]There is a difference between Chinese, Korean, and American ginseng. This recipe only uses American ginseng because of this difference.

Bone Soup

INGREDIENTS:

> 1½ pounds marrow bones
> ½ cup oil
> 5 small to medium-sized potatoes, cut into cubes
> 8–12 small plum tomatoes, cut into pieces
> ½–1 medium-sized fennel bulb, chopped
> Pinch or two of cinnamon
> ½ cup red wine (optional)
> 5–6 cups water
> Salt to taste

Be creative and use other vegetables such as carrots, celery, scallions, etc.

DIRECTIONS:
1. Rinse bones and set aside.
2. In a 4–5-quart stock pot, sauté the potatoes, tomato, and fennel along with any other vegetables of your choice in oil.
3. Add bones, water, wine, and spices and bring to a boil.
4. Reduce heat and simmer for several hours, stirring occasionally.

Three-Green Sauté

INGREDIENTS:

> Approximately 1 pound greens: ⅓ pound each broccoli rabe, chicory, and dandelion greens
> 2 quarts water
> 1 tablespoon walnut or other light oil
> 1 teaspoon salt
> 2 large cloves garlic, minced
> ½ teaspoon ginger root, minced

1 cup sliced mushrooms
1 tablespoon pine nuts, toasted (in walnut or other light oil)
$^1/_2$ teaspoon cinnamon

DIRECTIONS:

1. Wash greens, trim, and remove spoiled leaves.
2. Chop greens into 4-inch pieces.
3. Bring water to a boil; add greens and reduce heat.
4. Cook for 2 minutes; remove greens and set aside.
5. In a preheated wok or large heavy skillet, add oil and heat until it is very hot.
6. Add salt, garlic, and ginger (do not brown).
7. Quickly add the mushrooms and sauté until the juices begin to release.
8. Add greens, stir well, and cook until heated thoroughly.
9. Turn out on a serving dish and sprinkle with cinnamon and pine nuts.

Sweet and Sour Vegetable Stir-Fry

INGREDIENTS:

2 tablespoons walnut oil
$^1/_2$ cup scallion greens, diced
2 teaspoons garlic, minced
3 teaspoons fresh ginger, minced
2 cups broccoli florets
1 cup carrots, sliced
1 cup tomatoes, diced
1 cup mushrooms, sliced
1 cup snow pea pods
$^1/_2$ cup water chestnuts, diced
1 teaspoon cornstarch
$^1/_4$ cup cold water
$^1/_2$ cup soy sauce
2 tablespoons honey
2 tablespoons lemon juice

DIRECTIONS:

1. In a preheated wok or large heavy skillet, heat oil.
2. Add the scallions and stir-fry until they wilt and then add the garlic and ginger.
3. Add the broccoli and carrots; stir-fry until they begin to sweat.
4. Add the tomatoes, mushrooms, snow pea pods, and water chestnuts.
5. Mix the cornstarch into the cold water and add into the soy sauce, honey, and lemon juice.
6. Add the mixture to the vegetables and stir-fry until done.

Party-Dressed Snow Peas

INGREDIENTS:

2 tablespoons walnut oil
2 tablespoons scallion greens, chopped
1 clove garlic, crushed
1/2 teaspoon salt
1/4 teaspoon ground black pepper
4 bell peppers—2 red, 2 yellow, diced
1/2 cup white wine (optional)
1 pound snow pea pods

DIRECTIONS:

1. In a preheated wok or large, heavy skillet, heat the oil over medium heat.
2. Add the scallions, garlic, salt, and black pepper.
3. When the scallions begin to wilt, add the bell peppers and stir-fry for about 5 minutes, just before the pepper color really brightens.
4. Add the wine and snow pea pods and stir-fry for about 3 minutes; when the pea pods are a bright green, they are done.

Fruit Salad

INGREDIENTS:

> ²/₃ cup orange juice
> 2 cinnamon sticks
> ³/₄ cup strawberries, sliced
> 1 cup peaches, sliced
> ¹/₂ pear, cored and sliced
> ¹/₂ apple, cored and sliced
> ¹/₂ cup pineapple, chopped
> 1 banana, sliced
> ¹/₄ teaspoon nutmeg

DIRECTIONS:

1. Bring orange juice to a boil, put in cinnamon sticks, reduce heat, cover, and cook for 6 minutes.
2. Place all fruit in a bowl and pour the cooked juice over it; remove cinnamon sticks.
3. Toss together well and sprinkle nutmeg over the top. Cover and refrigerate for at least 2 hours.

CHAPTER 13

THE DRAGON'S WAY:
Most Frequently Asked Questions

ABOUT THE *WU MING* MERIDIAN THERAPY

Q. *Are these movements designed to burn calories?*
A. Burning calories is a side benefit of practicing *Wu Ming* Meridian Therapy Qigong movements. These are very ancient energy movements, which I have developed with my own master, Professor Xihua Xu of Yunnan, China. Professor Xu is a Qigong grand master and has worked at the highest level of the Chinese government. His specialty is Qigong for medical and healing purposes. Each movement has a special purpose and has the power to unblock Qi in your meridians or the energy pathways that run through your body and connect all of its internal structures. When your Qi strengthens, you will burn calories automatically and more efficiently. The more you have a good quality practice, the more you will benefit.

Q. *What is the best time to practice?*
A. The best time to practice is when you feel fresh, happy, and relaxed. Many people find that doing these ten Dragon's Way movements in the morning before they begin their day works

best. It's also a good idea to practice at the same time each day. In the beginning, try to do the entire set of ten movements more than once a day. Twice is the best, but remember, quality is better than quantity.

Q. *What do you mean by good quality?*
A. Good quality means during your practice your body, mind, and spirit work together as one holistic system. Every time you practice, try to feel the Qi flowing freely through your meridians and organs. After you practice, you should feel that you have a lot of energy throughout your day, that you feel less hungry, that you can handle stress better than before, and that you can sleep well. You may even notice that some chronic health problem that used to bother you has lessened dramatically.

Q. *Is there a special way to breathe during Qigong practice?*
A. The ability to regulate breathing for various activities is a natural skill that we are born with. These Qigong movements can strengthen this particular skill. Therefore, your breathing will automatically match each movement's needs. I never instruct my students on how to breathe. I like to make a joke with them. I say, "When you were born, your mother didn't give you breathing lessons, did she?" Everything about our *Wu Ming* Meridian Therapy is in concert with the natural law. This is not supposed to be an "effort." It is supposed to restore you. As the quality of your Qi changes, your breathing will automatically change as well. Don't hold your breath. Just listen to your body and follow what it wants to do naturally. It is not necessary to worry about whether you are breathing "correctly." Remember, the best technique is no technique.

Q. *Is it good to practice with my eyes closed?*
A. I recommend that you practice only *The Dragon Stands Between Heaven and Earth* (#10) with your eyes closed. For the other movements, you should practice with your eyes open so

that you can train your mind to practice in harmony with your body.

Q. *What should I focus on or think about when I practice* Wu Ming *Meridian Therapy?*
A. There are two general ways of approaching the answer to this question. The first follows the ancient Chinese saying: "If you can't control something, let it go." The mind is going to think, so why worry about it? Just let it go where it will. Eventually, with practice, you will find that the *Wu Ming* Meridian Therapy itself will cut off your thoughts and help you move to a calmer, more peaceful place where you can truly touch what is eternal within you. The rewards of continual practice are very great. If you find it difficult to let your thoughts go, then try another approach, which is to visualize the kind of body you want, how many pounds and inches you wish to give up, and how you will look in six weeks. As you perform each movement, imagine how it can bring you closer to your special goal.

Q. *Can you supplement the* Wu Ming *Meridian Therapy with other forms of exercise, such as walking, swimming, and weight lifting?*
A. There are many different types of walking; however, the only one that is truly beneficial is walking like old people. That is, you should walk very slowly and casually. Or you can go to a park and sit and listen to the birds, look at the trees and flowers. This is both helpful and healthful. It also gives you a special chance to connect with and receive the support of the Qi that is abundant in nature. You may not experience mature Qi with your mind, but your body will know that it is there. And it is there for you to tap into and get rejuvenated.

Swimming is a excellent exercise, especially if you swim for pleasure. Competitive swimming, or racing—even yourself—is not as good for you. Remember, our bodies are about 70 percent water. Water-type bodies benefit most from slow, flowing, water-type exercises.

The purpose of weight lifting is to build muscle mass. If you look at a cat, it has very sleek muscles and a lot of strength and spring to its movements. If you look at a cow, you see that it has a lot of muscle mass and not a lot of strength and spring to its movements. Which would you prefer to be like—a cow or a cat? From my martial arts training I have learned that strength, speed, and flexibility come from the tendon, and not the muscle.

Remember, if you can run, you can walk; if you can walk, you can stand; if you can stand, you can sit; and if you can sit, you can do nothing. And, from the Taoist point of view, nothing is truly everything. Think about this!

Q. *When I practice* The Dragon Stands Between Heaven and Earth *(#10), I get very tired. Shouldn't I stop at this point?*
A. No! In this Qigong system, this is precisely when you must push yourself. When you get shaky or tired while practicing *The Dragon Stands Between Heaven and Earth* (#10), this is the point at which your body is starting to increase its Qi. The longer you can practice this movement, the more Qi you can accumulate. Though you many not think so, these signs are positive ones. It is important to push yourself beyond this phase. You will pass through it and you will not always feel this uncomfortable. Unlike Western exercises, this is an energy situation that indicates your Qi is trying to push itself through your meridians for healing and weight loss. Be kind and be patient with yourself. Try to push through this feeling. Even if you only increase your time by a few seconds a day, you have opened the right door and are on the right path.

Q. *How do I know if my body is benefiting from* Wu Ming *Meridian Therapy?*
A. If after you practice, you sigh, yawn, or stretch, these are indicators of an internal benefit. So is feeling energized or sim-

ply relaxed. Some people do not "feel" anything special and yet are receiving tremendous benefit. Other people may "feel" a lot and yet their benefit may not be as great. In my classes, I recommend that Dragon's Way participants try not to look for quick results. The benefits from these movements may be readily apparent to some people and only show up over a longer period of practice time for others. Each of us is unique, and each of us will respond to the energy differently. If you are doing The Dragon's Way with a partner, do not compare your results or even your experiences. The amazing long-range healing effects of these movements will only appear over a period of time as these movements become the bedrock of your new life.

Q. *Do I really need to practice* Wu Ming *Meridian Therapy every day?*
A. Yes, it is critical to stress that the *Wu Ming* Meridian Therapy is the most important part of our program. If you've been a regular at exercise programs, or you are a veteran of many diet programs, you will most likely focus on the foods and the "eating for healing" information as the power source for The Dragon's Way. But this is not the right place to look. The true power and efficacy comes from the *Wu Ming* Meridian Therapy Qigong. These unique movements will help you increase your Qi and provide you with an internal energy cleansing. The best example I can give is that doing these movements is the equivalent of taking a daily shower for your internal organs and meridians. At least once during the day, take the time, about twenty minutes, to do all of the movements. I strongly recommend that you continue to do these healing movements after the six-week program and make them part of your life. You will continue to experience amazing benefits.

ABOUT QI

Q. *What do you mean when you talk about Qi or vital energy?*
A. Qi is the life force that animates everything in the Universe. It also animates your entire body and all its structures. It has two aspects: one is energy, or the power that drives a particular function, the second is information, or the right message. Of these two, information is more important than energy. If you have a simple Qi problem, usually you can solve it by taking a rest or eating certain foods, taking a vacation, or practicing some kind of meditation. It is when your Qi becomes unbalanced, through stress, illness, or disease, that vague problems like headaches or stomachaches begin to appear. These are warning signs that something internal needs to be fixed. If left untreated, these symptoms can often progress to more serious ones.

Q. *What happens if a Qi problem becomes worse?*
A. Let me answer with an example. Every day at 3:00 P.M. you get a headache. Then, without taking anything, it disappears at 3:30 P.M. You have undergone many different tests and you've been told that all your scientific tests indicate that there is no problem. The doctors say you are fine. You, however, know for certain that you are not fine, because every day at 3:00 P.M. you still get a headache that lasts for half an hour. You are not imagining this pain. It is very real. TCM would immediately identify this headache as a problem of unbalanced Qi. The Qi that flows through one of the six major meridians that run up through your head is blocked at some point along the way. This Qi blockage then causes your headache pain. There is no scientifically detectable source or disease yet. The headache is a symptom or a message from your body telling you that one or more of your organs is out of balance and not in harmony with the others. If you always experience a headache across your forehead, your stomach Qi is out of balance. If you have pain on either side of your head, you should look to the gallbladder.

Headaches that occur at the top of the head relate to the kidney or liver. The location of any headache is of utmost importance to a TCM practitioner; the time of day is also essential for a proper diagnosis. In this case, the organ that is "on duty" in the body from 1:00 P.M. to 3:00 P.M. is the small intestine. If your headache occurs at this time with regularity, it means that your small intestine is suffering from a Qi dysfunction. If you get heartburn or develop palpitations during this time period, TCM recognizes that these symptoms are related to the heart, but they have their origins in a small intestine Qi disorder. Be careful: this organ is sending you a very important message.

Q. *What is the difference between physical energy and internal Qi?*
A. Physical energy has its limits, while internal Qi is limitless because of its ability to access Universal Qi. Through *Wu Ming* Meridian Therapy, you can actually tap into the Qi of the Universe and connect with an endless, unbounded sea of unconditional love and energy. That is why The Dragon's Way is unique. It offers you something no other weight management program or weight control product can. It offers you the opportunity of a lifetime to heal for a lifetime. I hope that you will truly take advantage of the ancient wisdom and knowledge in The Dragon's Way.

ABOUT EATING

Q. *Are there specific quantities or specific times of the day to eat?*
A. Because everyone is different, The Dragon's Way has no specific quantities or measurements to recommend for eating. The best advice I can give you is that you should eat only until you feel about 70 percent full. The amount of food that can create a feeling of being 70 percent full will vary not only from person to person, but from day to day for the same person. Your whole body is a highly sensitive feedback system. What I would like you to learn is how to understand and really tune in to

what it wants and what makes it feel healthy. Remember do not eat a big meal late at night and then go to sleep. If you do, your body will expend Qi throughout the night just to digest this meal. This is Qi you need to conserve to help yourself heal the root cause of your excess weight. When it's late and you are hungry, drink something warm such as tea—even a cup of soup will help you. Have a few roasted walnuts or eat fruit.

Q. *Am I supposed to eat only the foods of The Dragon's Way for the rest of my life?*
A. No. This is The Dragon's Way Eating for Healing plan of recommended foods. Each and every one of the foods and condiments has been selected based on TCM theory for their ability to heal a specific organ related to weight problems. They are only recommendations for now and are intended to cleanse your body and give it a rest from the foods you normally eat and the eating patterns that you have lived by. After these six weeks of The Dragon's Way, like so many of our participants, you will know better how to take care of yourself and listen to your intuition. You will have learned how to use these and other foods for self-healing. After these six weeks, you may include other foods.

Q. *What foods can I eat?*
A. I want to emphasize the value of eating fresh foods. I strongly suggest that you stop eating foods with preservatives, additives, chemicals, genetically altered material, or false nutrients (nutrients that have been added into the food). One of the goals of this program is to help you learn how to listen to your intuition in choosing foods that support your health. If you learn well, you will reactivate your ability to discriminate between which foods are fresh and which are not.

Q. *Will I feel hungry on this program?*
A. You might experience some hunger because your regular patterns of eating have changed. But this is not a restrictive

food control program. If you feel hungry, you can use the Reverse Breathing Exercise for increasing Qi and eliminating hunger in Chapter 2, or you can eat something on the Eating for Healing recommended list. Having a warm drink, such as Chinese herbal tea or clear soup, can also help.

Q. *In the past when I have eaten primarily fruits and vegetables, I have become exceedingly tired and not been able to complete the diet because I would just not feel well. When I look at the foods you recommend, it seems like the same thing. Should I do this program?*
A. Your previous condition definitely makes sense. Your body did not have the Qi or energy support to function properly. The critical difference in The Dragon's Way is our *Wu Ming* Meridian Therapy, which will give you the energy support that you need to build internal strength so that you can maintain an Eating for Healing plan without feeling the conditions you mentioned. The more you practice these ancient healing Qigong movements, the better and stronger you will feel. Also, your body will be able to use food more efficiently.

Q. *Can I eat vegetables other than those on the Recommended Foods for Healing list?*
A. Yes. But you will get the best results from The Dragon's Way by choosing your foods primarily (if not totally) from the Recommended Foods for Healing list. Each and every one of the foods has been chosen for a healing purpose. The more of them that you eat, the more healing benefit you will derive. Remember, we are working at healing the root cause of your weight problem. We are working at rebalancing the organs responsible for the weight maintenance mechanisms in your body. At long last, you're really dealing with the cause of your weight problem, not the symptom. Be patient, but be glad. If you can truly heal the source of the problem, you also won't experience the rebound effect that discourages and frustrates so many dieters.

I always tell my students and participants, "Eat what your body tells you it wants." If you go out to eat, challenge yourself. Order the foods available using your intuition, which should keep you far away from fried or barbecued foods!

Q. *Can I have vegetables for lunch and fruit for dinner?*
A. Yes.

Q. *Can I have both vegetables and fruit for both dinner and lunch?*
A. Yes.

Q. *Is it better to eat cooked or raw vegetables?*
A. During The Dragon's Way, this is one of my most important recommendations: Do not eat raw vegetables. I understand that when vegetables are cooked they can lose a little vitamins and nutrition, but we are looking beyond food's physical properties, to its energy dimension. If you continually eat raw vegetables and cold salads, your body will use up more energy or healing Qi to digest them. You will also eventually unbalance your stomach's function.

After vegetables are cooked, even lightly, they will be easier to digest. That is the major thing. Also, remember that according to the natural law, your stomach doesn't like cold foods or drinks, or foods with a cold essence. It prefers foods that are warm or have a warm essence. Switching to these foods and drinks alone will help improve your digestion immensely. You may be very surprised at how different this makes you feel.

Q. *Can I use a microwave oven for cooking?*
A. Yes, you can. However, try this test. Heat one cup of milk on the stove and another cup of milk in the microwave. Then put both cups on a table or counter and see which one will turn sour first. Usually, it is the milk from the microwave. Experiment by doing this with other foods. You'll see that it is the

microwaved food that most often spoils first because the natural structure of the food has been destroyed.

Q. *Can I cook food in advance?*
A. Yes. There is nothing wrong with doing this and reheating your food later. Try to use the oven or top of the stove instead of a microwave, if possible. Given our busy lifestyles, it's important to be practical in following The Dragon's Way. Whenever possible, however, try to eat fresh, cooked foods.

Q. *Can I drink coffee and tea? If so, can I use milk, half-and-half, sugar or artificial sweeteners?*
A. Yes, you can still drink tea and coffee on The Dragon's Way. The program isn't trying to take anything away from you, especially if you love it. You also may continue to use sugar, milk, and half-and-half. I recommend that you use real sugar instead of artificial sweeteners. For one thing, artificial sweeteners have a taste that is many times sweeter than sugar or honey. This conditions your mouth and mind to a taste level that is much sweeter than what you would naturally eat. For another thing, focusing on a tiny packet of sweetener in the belief that it will really help you deal with the root cause of weight problems is not productive or realistic. What will help you is changing your daily habits as we've outlined in this book. I also recommend that you drink milk and half-and-half in moderation. Many participants also ask me if it's all right to drink skim milk or low-fat milk. I ask them, "Do cows give skim milk or low-fat milk?" I prefer that you drink milk that has not been processed to create these products. You are better off drinking whole milk products. The same is true for butter; I prefer that you eat real butter and avoid low-fat substitutes and margarine.

Q. *How much water should I drink?*
A. First of all, I recommend that you do not drink eight glasses of water a day. I suggest you drink only when you are thirsty. Don't carry bottles of water around with you all the time. You

are simply conditioning yourself to drink water all day long. According to TCM, drinking large amounts of water uses excess kidney Qi and puts a strain on your bladder as well. Your bladder also has to power up to process the excess water, and its Qi too is used up faster. One of the ideas I would like you to learn from The Dragon's Way is that you will have tremendous long-term health benefits by conserving your kidney's Inborn Qi.

Q. *Is honey better than white sugar?*
A. Yes. Honey is a natural antibiotic and its warming essence is good for supporting the energy of your lung and large intestine.

Q. *Can I eat eggs?*
A. Eat only the whites of eggs during The Dragon's Way; in fact, for the rest of your life. Eggs whites provide high protein. The yolks, as we all know, are high in cholesterol that requires the gallbladder to use more of its Qi or energy to process. The whole point of The Dragon's Way is to conserve as much Qi as possible to heal the root cause of excess weight. If you do choose to eat egg whites during the program, try to eat them at dinner. Quail eggs, if you can find them, offer much better Qi or energy than chicken or other kinds of eggs.

Q. *Where can I find some of the more unusual foods in the program?*
A. Almost all of the Foods for Healing recommended in this program are readily found in your regular grocery store or supermarket. Most of the food recommendations are common fruits, vegetables, spices, herbs, and oils. Special suggestions such as the quail eggs are not required. There are a few foods that are very healing that you can find in a Chinese grocery store. I think most large cities have at least one or two of these.

Q. *Should I eat only organic fruits and vegetables? Are they better?*
A. If you can readily obtain organic food at reasonable prices, this is definitely better for you. From the TCM point of view,

it is important to understand that it is the internal function of your organs that must be kept strong. Then they can defend you from external pathogens. Focusing externally only on specific foods is not the answer.

Q. *If I eat pine nuts rather than walnuts, how many do I eat?*
A. Pine nuts are very filling and quite rich, so I think a small handful should be enough. Again, you should pay attention to your body and not your mind. Try to feel if you're really hungry or if you just want to eat more pine nuts—either because they taste so good, or perhaps you're emotionally out of sorts and you want to keep on eating something.

Q. *Can I substitute another nut for the walnuts or pine nuts in the morning?*
A. Both walnuts and pine nuts have a very strong kind of energy essence that other nuts cannot match. They are especially effective for boosting your kidney Qi. You can also eat cashews and almonds during the program. You should always toast any nuts before eating or cooking with them because it conserves your Qi for healing and makes them easier to digest.

Q. *What is the benefit of toasting the walnuts?*
A. They are easier to digest and heating them brings out their essence.

Q. *I am allergic to some nuts. What do I do for protein?*
A. Try pine nuts. See if they work for you. If not, just do not eat the nuts for the first few weeks. From the TCM point of view, food allergies are due to a digestive imbalance. Therefore, as your digestive system heals and you strengthen your Qi, you will find that your food allergies might simply disappear. If not, you can include cooked egg whites instead of the nuts.

Q. *Do I have to eat three meals a day or can I do something like have the walnuts in the morning and then a piece of fruit an hour or so later followed by more fruit in another hour, and so on?*

A. The whole idea of The Dragon's Way is to educate you and help you learn how to listen to *your* body, not to me. Remember, I want you to have the gift of a lifetime, for a lifetime. Your body is smart and can heal itself if you support it in its efforts. If you've been out of balance for a while, you must understand that to truly heal, you should consider this effort a long-term process. There are no "quick fixes" for regaining your health. You must do the work, not just today and tomorrow, but every day. Eat in a way that accommodates what your body tells you it needs to eat and when it needs to eat.

Q. *Should the juices I select be fresh-squeezed rather than commercial products?*

A. Fresh juice is always better. It's especially important to drink fresh juice during the six weeks of the program so that your body will learn the difference between fresh juice and commercially processed products.

Q. *Why is watermelon juice so important?*

A. Watermelon is a remarkable fruit and has been prescribed by TCM practitioners for a variety of conditions for many centuries. Because its energy essence helps to reduce internal heat, it is good for digestion and acts as a diuretic. It also has the ability to remove toxins from the body. Other melons do not have the same healing properties.

Q. *Why do you recommend avoiding cheese during the program?*

A. Cheese causes the stomach to overwork. Remember, some of the foods on the list have been selected because they are gentle on your digestive system, which, in turn, helps you conserve your Qi for healing the root cause of your excess weight.

Q. *What about fish and seafood?*
A. After the program, fish and seafood are excellent foods to add back into your eating plan and are definitely a better choice than meat. Because they come from the "salty" sea, in most cases, they are good for helping support kidney function (whose taste in The Five Element Theory Chart is salty). If you find yourself invited to a party during this program where the best shrimp and fish are served, don't pass them up! Just make sure you practice more the next day.

Q. *Can I use onions rather than scallions?*
A. No. Scallions have a healing Qi that onions don't have. If you must use onions for some reason, then red onions are the best.

Q. *Can I eat yogurt?*
A. I do not recommend that you eat yogurt of any kind during The Dragon's Way program. Yogurt is not only cold in and of itself, but it also has a cold essence, which I would like you to eliminate or avoid as much as possible. You will save a lot of Qi by doing this.

Q. *What about seaweed?*
A. Seaweed is very good for your thyroid function. Sometimes, a person doesn't lose weight because his/her thyroid is not functioning properly. Remember, even if you've been tested for a thyroid problem and been told that it is fine, it is possible that its function is out of balance with the rest of your organs. This kind of function problem or Qi imbalance would not show up on scientific tests, but would be apparent through a TCM pulse diagnosis.

Q. *I have many food allergies. What should I do?*
A. Most people in the West believe that any health problems they have are caused by factors that are outside of their own body. But think about this: If we went to a party and asked

fifteen people if they had a wheat allergy, you might be the only one. Why? It's not the wheat that's the problem, it's your body's inability to process it appropriately. The food is not the problem. The TCM point of view on food allergies is that they originate with an imbalance in the digestive system. As you coax your spleen/stomach partnership back into balance, help your organs function and get Qi flowing more freely again, you should find that your allergy symptoms abate or disappear.

Q. *Can I drink alcohol during this program?*
A. Yes you can, but not every day. If one or two glasses of wine or bottles of beer makes you happy, then go ahead. If you feel sick, nauseous, or wake up with a headache the next day, you should recognize that The Dragon's Way is causing internal changes. Pay attention to these signals; listen to your body and not your mind. I do not recommend drinking hard liquor during the program

Q. *After the program is over, what meat can I eat and still help my organs function properly?*
A. After the program, after you feel you have rebalanced your digestive system, eat whatever you want. Listen to your body, not your mind. Here is some TCM information about a few meats you might find interesting: venison is considered to be best for the kidney; quail and quail eggs are good for the lung; lamb is better than beef; wild duck is good for arthritis. If possible, I recommend that you avoid eating too much red meat.

Q. *I'm concerned about getting enough calcium while I am on this program because there are no dairy foods.*
A. Ingesting calcium, even on a regular basis, does not necessarily mean that you are actually receiving its benefits. According to TCM, if your digestive system is unbalanced and not functioning properly, you cannot fully absorb the nutrients from the food you eat or supplements you ingest. Or, for that matter,

from anything else that you put into your stomach. And so, for the initial six-week period while you are training your body, I recommend that you do not eat hard-to-digest foods, many of which are high in calcium. When your digestive system improves and begins to function properly, your body will absorb calcium and other nutrients more fully. Furthermore, some of the foods in The Dragon's Way, such as broccoli, do provide calcium.

ABOUT THE BODY

Q. *What does TCM consider the #1 cause of excess weight?*
A. Stress, stress, and stress! Remember, stress affects the way your liver functions. In order for your digestive system to work well, your stomach/spleen, kidney/urinary bladder, liver/gallbladder, and lung/large intestine must function effectively in and of themselves, and they must work harmoniously in one interconnected system.

The tension we retain because of stress reduces the flow of Qi throughout the body. Consequently, each organ suffers individually and their partnership with their companion organ also suffers. Stress also causes you to go into your kidney's energy saving account and deplete the amount of irreplaceable Inborn Qi that you were born with. Stress is a serious enemy and you should treat it as such. Do not underestimate the harm stress can do. If you are overweight, look to the many areas in your life where you can reduce stress and become more peaceful. I promise you, you will be saving your own life

Q. *How can I tell if my stomach is hot or has a condition of excess heat?*
A. Generally speaking, if your stomach has a condition of excess internal heat, you might have bad breath or a bitter kind of taste in your mouth virtually all the time. Most likely, you will also be constipated. Sometimes individuals with excess heat in

the stomach also have constipation and/or acne on their forehead or near their nose. Sometimes they also exhibit a red nose.

Q. *I am experiencing a kind of itching just under my skin during The Dragon's Way. What is this?*
A. It is not unusual for some people to experience a certain kind of itching sensation during The Dragon's Way. This happens when there is an increase of Qi flowing through the meridians, or energy channels, which connect all the body's structures. Other people experience a tingling sensation. Often these feelings seem to travel around the body. For some, the itching or tingling is localized to a specific area. This is your own healing Qi beginning to move through your body. This is a positive sign that Qi is beginning to flow.

Q. *During the first several days of the program, I have been experiencing a lot of gas. What does this mean?*
A. Generally speaking, this means that your body is going through an internal Qi cleansing. If you have gas without a strong odor, this means that your internal organs are pretty clean. If your gas has a very strong smell, then you are getting rid of internal toxins. This is a positive sign. After the program, you can use this body sign to tell if the foods you're eating are good for you. For instance, if you eat meat, a lot of dairy foods or heavy protein, your gas might have a bad odor. Generally speaking, fresh fruits and vegetables do not cause gas with a strong odor.

Q. *I have been experiencing bloating. What does this mean?*
A. Most often, stomach distension means that your liver and stomach are not functioning in harmony with each other. The organs themselves may be fine, but the way they are performing their assigned tasks is not. As you continue with the program, this should gradually go away. Try to practice *Wu Ming* Meridian Therapy Qigong movements as frequently as you can.

Q. *I have experienced some leg muscle cramps at night. What should I do?*

A. Cramps in your leg muscles at night means that your bladder is suffering from a condition of excess cold. Add more spicy foods like cinnamon and ginger to the meals you eat during the day. Each night before you go to bed, take a hot bath or soak your feet above your ankles in very warm water. Another thing you can do is rub the bottoms of your feet until they are very warm. This should help.

Q. *I have been carefully following the program for about five weeks and I am noticing that my sense of taste and smell are sharper. Am I imagining this?*

A. This is one normal and highly positive effect of The Dragon's Way. As your internal organs heal, the sensory organs associated with them improve as well. Study The Five Element Theory Chart in Chapter 6 and notice which sensory organs are the "window" of which organ. Whenever something changes, identify it to yourself. This is part of the self-healing process. You may want to write about this improvement in your Healing Journal. Acknowledge yourself for awakening your special gift.

Q. *I'm pleased to say that I've lost inches as well as pounds during this program. I have lost more inches than the pounds would indicate and yet I am not working out. Can you explain this?*

A. Because your Qi is now moving more freely, your body has become firmer and has rid itself of excess water. After eliminating water, the body then goes on to eliminate fat. Also, a Qigong practice has more benefit than a workout session. You might notice that your physical strength, body balance, joint flexibility, and posture all improve tremendously.

Q. *I have come down with a cold while doing The Dragon's Way. What can I do?*

A. When you have a cold, you have a Qi deficiency. To treat your cold's root cause, it's then necessary to increase Qi. I suggest that you sit down, close your eyes and meditate, which can recharge your Qi. Also, if you experience a cold, try practicing a set of the *Wu Ming* Meridian Therapy Qigong movements. You can also try drinking ginger tea. Make yourself a special tea from fresh ginger slices, the diced white part of scallions and brown sugar. Boil the ginger and the diced white part of the scallions in several cups of water. Strain and add brown sugar to taste. Take a really warm shower and get into bed under the covers. You might find that you can push this cold energy out of your body naturally without taking any over-the-counter medications.

Q. *I seem to have reached a plateau in my weight loss. The past two or three weeks I have been the same weight. Is there anything you can suggest to get beyond this plateau?*
A. Be patient. Although you may have reached a plateau with other weight loss programs, The Dragon's Way is very different. Your body probably just needs a rest. Even if you are not losing weight, your internal organs systems are getting stronger. Things are happening deep beneath the surface, little things are beginning to happen.

Be patient, trust yourself. Your internal systems need to accumulate enough Qi to prepare for the next breakthrough. If you start worrying, you can set yourself up for undoing the good work you've already done. Remember that the spleen's emotion is anxiety or overthinking. Also, I do not recommend that participants weigh themselves frequently during The Dragon's Way because I do not want them to confuse weight loss with true healing. Though you may lose many pounds, you may not be completely healed and may stop this important processing.

ABOUT THE PROGRAM

Q. *Why are some weeks of The Dragon's Way harder than others?*
A. This varies with each person. Because The Dragon's Way is a self-healing program, each week you are dealing with different levels of healing. In general, change is difficult, and when your body is starting to change, you are challenged to push yourself through it in order to gain the benefits. A healthy, balanced body maintains its normal weight naturally, without strenuous exercises, drastic diets, or crazy lifestyle habits. It does not gain and retain excess weight. If you have this condition, your body is not healthy or balanced. It takes work to recover and regain your healing abilities. Be patient with yourself. You are now dealing with the root cause.

Q. *This is only a six-week program. How do I maintain my health gains and weight loss after The Dragon's Way?*
A. During the course of this program you have been practicing what you will hopefully do for the rest of your life, such as nurturing and enhancing your self-healing ability; conserving Qi; avoiding stress; listening to your body's needs; choosing what you eat carefully; and above all, practicing *Wu Ming* Meridian Therapy. Think of *Wu Ming* Meridian Therapy as an internal shower that you can take to help you clean up any physical or emotional Qi stagnation accumulated during your day. You can use this program for a few days each week or several times a month to prevent health problems and avoid regaining weight. Remember, health is not a destination: it's a way of life.

Q. *Do you recommend fasting?*
A. For some people, I would say, absolutely not! For others, I might say try it. It depends on your present physical and emotional condition. Fasting means you push your body to a certain level and then the body itself can change inside. If someone is

very healthy, fasting offers some benefits for cleansing the body. For this program, you will gain many more benefits from increasing your Qi than pushing yourself to the limit. This is especially true if you have a lot of weight to lose, or if you have other health conditions.

Q. *I eat out in restaurants a lot. During The Dragon's Way, do I have to change my lifestyle?*
A. Not really. Almost all restaurants have vegetarian meals and vegetable dishes with things like broccoli and cauliflower. Fresh fruit is usually available as well. Many have good soups (not the kind with cream). If you ask, they also will bring you hot tea instead of ice water at the beginning of the meal. If you're really hungry, it's fine to eat a little bread or breadsticks.

Q. *I am interested in losing weight, but I am also interested in lowering cholesterol. How does the program work with that?*
A. As their healing abilities strengthen and their organs begin to function better, many program participants have found that their cholesterol levels drop naturally over the course of the program. We've had many participants pleasantly surprise their doctors while on The Dragon's Way. Quite a few were able to work with their physicians, who readjusted or lowered their cholesterol medication.

Q. *I have a lot of allergies, especially food allergies. How will the program affect me?*
A. Through this program, you might find that your food allergies diminish and finally go away. I have seen this happen many times. Generally speaking, TCM regards food allergies as a stomach function disorder. This situation results when the liver overcontrols the stomach. When you change your diet and practice energy healing, you might find that when the function of these two important organs improves, your food allergies will get better. From the TCM perspective, the

food itself is not the problem. One of the goals of The Dragon's Way is to jumpstart the stomach and get it to function or perform its assigned tasks the way it should, thereby addressing the root cause of the allergies.

Q. *I have high blood pressure and I am taking medication. Does this present a problem?*
A. Before you embark on The Dragon's Way, advise your doctor about what you are doing. This program will not interfere with your medication. Neither will taking blood pressure medication prevent you from gaining the healing benefits of *Wu Ming* Meridian Therapy. Again, we've had quite a number of participants who have very pleasantly surprised their doctors with the positive effect this program has on normalizing blood pressure. In fact, in cooperation with their doctors, a number of participants have been able to either lower their dosage or eliminate their medication entirely. I believe you will definitely know during the program whether you are getting benefit from The Dragon's Way or not.

Q. *What about vitamins and nutritional supplements? Should I take them?*
A. During The Dragon's Way, I recommend that you take a minimal amount of vitamins or nutritional supplements. Allow your body to build up the strength of your digestive system with this self-healing program. When your digestive system is working well, you'll be able to get the vitamins you need from the food you eat. And, if you feel the need to continue taking vitamins after the program, you will be able to gain more benefit from them with a healthy digestive system. Listen to your body for what you need—not your mind, not the advertising agencies, not the media—but your own body.

Q. *I attend a lot of business functions. How can I adapt the principles of eating for energy to those situations?*

A. Be prepared! Most of the time you know in advance that you will be eating at a business function. Make sure ahead of time to take care of yourself in these situations. When you have the opportunity to choose from a menu, select warm foods such as soup. Don't drink the ice water that is often automatically served. Make the best choices that you can. Balance eating cold foods such as salad, with drinking tea, eating ginger or cooked fennel when you return home.

Q. *I am pregnant. Is this a good time for me to do this program?*
A. There are two parts to The Dragon's Way. While the Eating for Healing Plan is good for most people, pregnant women need to eat differently. However, the *Wu Ming* Meridian Therapy is good for everyone. If you practice Qigong during your pregnancy, your baby will automatically gain the benefits of this self-healing energy system. The best thing about practicing is that you will pass a very special gift that is beyond price to your unborn child. You will be putting extra Qi into her or his Inborn Savings Account. After you have your child, then The Dragon's Way can more fully help you to reawaken your healing ability, increase your Qi, cause it to flow smoothly throughout your meridians, and lose weight and inches naturally.

Q. *After the program is over, what should I eat?*
A. After the program, I believe you will have gained a fundamental healing benefit from The Dragon's Way. You will be able to listen to your body and not your mind. Your body should tell you what is good for you. In effect, you can eat whatever you like.

Q. *Are six weeks enough?*
A. Six weeks is enough time for most people's bodies to begin to function on a higher, more harmonious level. Some people just need a tune-up. Other people have a longer journey than

others; they need to do a lot more work. It depends on the state of your health and what your body needs when you start The Dragon's Way. I had a participant who unexpectedly stopped smoking and then after her body adjusted to not smoking, she lost weight. The root causes of weight problems are the same for almost everyone—an imbalance in the function of the liver, kidney, and spleen. This unique TCM theory-based program provides the information, tools and techniques to address these conditions and heal them for most people.

Acknowledgments

THE Dragon's Way Program has been running for nearly five years. By the time you read this book, close to one thousand participants will have gone through the program. It's been gratifying to see so many people derive so many benefits from traditional Chinese medicine and this self-healing plan. As individuals awaken their healing abilities, they are rewarded with better health than they ever expected. In addition to taking off weight and inches, we've seen individuals heal conditions—high blood pressure, high cholesterol, depression, migraines, hemorrhoids, digestive disturbances, to name a few—that have bothered them, in many cases, for more than a decade. Those of you who complete The Dragon's Way will see what I mean. The program benefits are extraordinary.

There are a number of people who deserve thanks for the roles they've played in helping The Dragon's Way become more widely known and the success that it is. First, I would like to give my deepest thanks to the participants in The Dragon's Way—to the brave individuals with a good heart who were willing to try something different. Your excitement, your challenges, your questions and your appreciation have strengthened

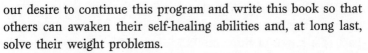

our desire to continue this program and write this book so that others can awaken their self-healing abilities and, at long last, solve their weight problems.

Louise DiBello, who manages The Dragon's Way for our Center, has put tremendous time and effort into making the program better and better each year. She has worked tirelessly to encourage people to open themselves up to the miracles of TCM. Her partner Kay Reynolds has also supported this program over the years. Kay's helpful questions and desire to make the program work for all the participants and address their needs is much appreciated. Along the way, there have been many instructors and volunteers at The Dragon's Way sessions who have unselfishly contributed their enthusiasm, as well as their time and effort. The gift of their energy and heart has always helped make the program a special one.

I would like to thank Ellasara Kling, who leaped without a backward glance into the challenging project of organizing the original Dragon's Way material. Without her special culinary skills, this book would not be as rich as it is in delicious, inventive recipes that can help participants stay with the program. Her intensive efforts to organize and test the recipes are deeply appreciated. Pat Snyder has once again lent us her considerable writing skills in pulling the material together into a book format. Pat's willingness to explore TCM deeper and deeper has made a major contribution to this book. And again, Karen Schulz has provided help by lending us her time and talent on graphics.

Without the intelligent organizational and editing efforts of Jennifer Brehl, senior editor at Avon Books, we would not have such a well-developed blueprint for The Dragon's Way. Her editing talent and insightful questions have helped sharpen the manuscript and make it more accessible. Our agent, Barbara Lowenstein, of Lowenstein & Associates, has been a constant in a very challenging project, always checking in to see how we are doing and giving us support and encouragement every step of the way.

Finally, I would like to thank my writing partner, Ellen Schaplowsky, for collaborating with me on this book, which is part of a series of three on TCM. Her drive and dedication to developing the finished work and to bringing this project to completion are appreciated beyond measure.

About Nan Lu, O.M.D., M.S., L.Ac.

*N*ᴬᴺ Lu, O.M.D., M.S., L.Ac., is the founder and president of the Traditional Chinese Medicine World Foundation and the American Taoist Healing Center, Inc., of New York and New Jersey. The nonprofit Foundation is the only facility of its kind dedicated to teaching *Wu Ming* Qigong in the United States. Dr. Lu is a classically trained doctor of TCM and a New York State licensed acupuncturist. His Foundation and Center are dedicated to serving as the source for authentic information on TCM and Taoist Qigong. The Foundation's mission is to build bridges of understanding between East and West in the areas of TCM, natural healing, and internal martial arts. Recently, the Foundation launched *Traditional Chinese Medicine World*, the first-ever newspaper to help educate consumers in the West about traditional Chinese medicine.

Dr. Lu began his training in China as a child in Taoist Qigong, TCM, and internal martial arts. Studying with several well-known, well-respected masters and doctors, he received special keys of understanding and the true essence of these ancient healing and internal martial arts, a privilege reserved for only the most advanced students. The unique healing knowledge

Dr. Lu has inherited cannot be found in medical textbooks. His extensive training is the kind that ancient doctors of TCM were expected to have so that they could understand the fundamental basis of TCM—how Qi moves through the body. As a Qigong master and international martial arts champion, Dr. Lu has refined his healing practice to a very high level.

An extraordinary martial artist, Dr. Lu has won many top honors. In the fall of 1997, he competed in Argentina in the Sixth International World Cup Championship, where he was named one of the top ten Taiji masters in the world. He has authored many columns for internal martial arts publications, including *Pa Kua Chang* Journal, *Wushu Kung Fu* and *Inside Kung Fu* magazines.

Dr. Lu is a member of the advisory group of participants for Columbia University's Center for Complementary & Alternative Medicine Research in Women's Health in a landmark study of Chinese herbs. He is also an advisory board member of the Transpersonal Psychology Association, the Hypoglycemia Support Foundation, and the USA Wushu Kungfu Federation. In New York, he works with SHARE, the self-help organization for women with breast or ovarian cancer. Through SHARE, Dr. Lu conducts a series of seminars where *Wu Ming* Qigong movements are taught to women with cancer to help them improve breast and ovarian health.

Dr. Lu holds a Doctorate in Traditional Chinese Medicine from Hubei College of Traditional Chinese Medicine, China, and a Master of Science degree from City University of New York (CUNY). He has authored numerous articles on TCM and Taoist Qigong. With his "Eastern Outlook" column for *Natural Way* magazine, Dr. Lu was the first-ever columnist on TCM for a major national health magazine. In 1999, he was named "Visionary of the Year" by the board of directors of the 3rd World Congress on Qigong and the 2nd American Qigong Conference. His practice includes the use of many herbal supplements based on ancient traditional Chinese formulas that he has developed and adapted for his Western patients. He has also developed a skin care treatment line based on TCM energy principles. Dr. Lu has lectured extensively on TCM, Qigong, and self-healing in China, the United States, and England.

About Ellen H. Schaplowsky

ELLEN Schaplowsky has more than twenty years of experience in marketing communications work for consumer products, and in reputation management and environmental marketing. She is an executive vice president of Ruder Finn, Inc., one of the world's largest independent public relations agencies, where she founded the company's "Marketing for the Environment" Group. The Group's mission is to help corporations, brand businesses, and nonprofit organizations communicate on complex issues so that practical solutions can be identified. As part of her work in this area, Ellen has served as a guest columnist for the *Earth Times*, the first global newspaper on issues of the environment and sustainability that emerged from the 1992 Earth Summit in Rio de Janeiro. She is also responsible for helping create and develop America's largest litter cleanup and recycling program, which annually attracts several million volunteers. For thirteen years, this program was conducted jointly by the GLAD® brand and Keep America Beautiful, Inc. It is regarded as one of the longest running partnerships in brand history.

During the early 1990s, Ellen was searching for an explanation and treatment for a complex of physical symptoms that no Western doctor seemed able to pinpoint and treat. After a number of years, she was diagnosed as having an autoimmune condition. It was at about the same time that she was introduced to the concept of Qi or "energy" practice and met Nan Lu. Ellen became Dr. Lu's patient and began a journey that would bring her deeper and deeper into TCM and its approach to self-healing and wellness. Eventually, she became a student at the American Taoist Healing Center and began practicing *Wu Ming* Qigong under the guidance of Dr. Lu.

While a patient and student, Ellen began applying her marketing communications skills to help Dr. Lu achieve his mission of serving as the authentic source for information on TCM and Taoist Qigong. At Dr. Lu's request, she became the vice president of the Center and consequently the Traditional Chinese Medicine World Foundation. In 1996, she and Dr. Lu began collaborating on writing the first-ever column on TCM for a national health magazine. After more than two years of developing this column, they embarked on a more ambitious writing project, the first version of what would become *Traditional Chinese Medicine: A Woman's Guide to Healing from Breast Cancer.* This collaboration marked their first book in a series of TCM works published by Avon Books. Ellen also serves as executive editor of the Foundation's newspaper, *Traditional Chinese Medicine World.*

About the Traditional Chinese Medicine World Foundation and the American Taoist Healing Center, Inc.

*T*HE American Taoist Healing Center, Inc., was founded in 1994 by Dr. Nan Lu. In the spring of 1999, it became part of the Traditional Chinese Medicine World Foundation, which operates as a nonprofit organization. Its mission is to build bridges of understanding between East and West through educational programs and services in the areas of Taoist Qigong, TCM, natural healing, and internal martial arts. The Foundation is dedicated to serving as the source for authentic information on traditional Chinese medicine and Taoist Qigong.

PROGRAMMING

TCM Treatment

Dr. Lu maintains a practice in New York City and Bloomfield, New Jersey. He uses Taoist Qigong, acupressure, acupuncture (in NYC), moxibustion, classical herbs, and Chinese medical massage to treat a variety of conditions. Areas of specialty include women's health, especially breast cancer, PMS, menopause, menstrual irregularities, chronic fatigue syndrome, arthritis, hay fever, allergies, tendonitis, and sports injuries as well as weight problems, to name a few. The focus of his practice is on preventing illness and disease, as well as helping patients heal themselves.

Wu Ming *Qigong*

Wu Ming Qigong is the basis for all programming at the Traditional Chinese Medicine World Foundation, the American Taoist Healing Center and Dr. Lu's medical practice. This unique self-healing energy system has never before been taught in the United States. It descends directly from the ancient Taoist masters Lao Tzu and Chuang Tzu. This special self-healing energy practice, which is easy to learn and produces results rapidly, helps students (and patients) connect their body, mind, spirit and emotions for maximum healing benefit. *Wu Ming* Qigong is taught in beginner and advanced levels.

Qigong Meridian Therapy (QMT)

The American Taoist Healing Center conducts training in Qigong Meridian Therapy (QMT) for therapists, which includes a grounding in the fundamentals of TCM and Taoist Qigong, as well as intensive training in special hand techniques for this medical treatment. QMT practitioners are certified jointly with the Center and Hubei College of TCM, Hubei, China. QMT practitioners have offered their services at a number of large firms and organizations, including Smith Barney, New York Department of Personnel, and the Mind/Body Medical Center of Morristown Hospital in New Jersey, among others.

The Dragon's Way

The Dragon's Way is the Traditional Chinese Medicine World Foundation's successful self-healing program for weight loss and stress management. It addresses the underlying factors causing weight problems in a seven-session program. The Dragon's Way uses the best of authentic TCM principles and theories to help individuals heal themselves and take off weight and inches. It combines *Wu Ming* Meridian Therapy, a special Eating for Healing Plan and TCM herbal formulas for maximum health. To date, close to one thousand individuals have gone through the program with excellent results. Participants lose an average of twelve pounds and eight inches. Most important are the reductions in health conditions like stress, high cholesterol, high blood pressure and the alleviation of other conditions like insomnia, food allergies, and stomach problems, to name a few.

Women's Health, Including PMS and Menopause Programs

The Foundation conducts programming for women's health that includes a special six-week course to help alleviate the symptoms of menopause, such as hot flashes, night sweats, insomnia, irritability, etc. TCM has been treating menopausal symptoms for thousands of years by addressing their common root cause— unbalanced liver Qi and kidney Qi deficiency. In fact, one famous herbal formula for hot flashes has been in use for centuries and is still used today in China. Dr. Lu has adapted this special formula for his Western menopause patients. This formulation is available through the Traditional Chinese Medicine World Foundation, whose address is in the back of this book.

The Breast Cancer Prevention Project

The Breast Cancer Prevention Project was launched in 1997 in New York City. Its mission is to bring the ancient self-healing knowledge of TCM and its centuries-old experience with breast cancer to as many women as possible. Recently, the Foundation began the Tamoxifen Program as part of the Breast Cancer Prevention Project. This seven-session program uses TCM principles and theories to treat the root cause of the menopausal symptoms caused by the anti-estrogenic agent tamoxifen. The Breast Cancer Prevention Project includes *Traditional Chinese Medicine: A Woman's Guide to Healing from Breast Cancer*, a companion video, outreach programs with organizations such as SHARE, the New York–based self-help organization for women with breast or ovarian cancer, and a website at www.breastcancer.com.

PRODUCTS

The following products have been developed by and are used by Dr. Nan Lu in his practice. They are based on TCM principles and theories.

- All-Natural Classical Chinese Herbal Food Supplements, adapated by Dr. Lu for The Dragon's Way. Includes *Imperial Qi* and *China Dirt*. They have been successfully used by close to one thousand program participants.
- All-Natural Classical Chinese Herbal Food Supplements, developed and adapted by Dr. Lu for a variety of health conditions, including:
  —The Breast Cancer Prevention Project BCPP Herbal Master line of herbs and natural herbal teas
  —Menopause Series of Classical Chinese Herbal Food Supplements
- All-Natural Herbal Skin Treatment Products
  —Acne Facial Masque: herbal masque helps correct underlying cause of acne
  —All Day/All Night Creme: stimulates meridians in the facial area and brings more nutrition into the face for a smoother, younger appearance
  —Silk Face Masque: a special all-natural combination of herbs that is blended with honey; helps pull toxins from the skin and creates a smooth, fresh-looking appearance.
- Videos
  —*Traditional Chinese Medicine for Weight Loss That Lasts*: The Dragon's Way practice video, a special real-

time session with Dr. Lu of all ten *Wu Ming* Meditation Therapy Qigong movements

—*Traditional Chinese Medicine for Today's Breast Cancer*, a video with Dr. Lu teaching *Wu Ming* Meridian Therapy movements. Features a real-time, twenty-minute practice session with Dr. Lu.

• Audiotapes:

—*The Dragon's Way*, A special real-time practice tape with Dr. Lu that helps participants go through a twenty-minute session of all ten *Wu Ming* Meditation Therapy Qigong movements. Side B features a half hour of Dr. Lu's "energy" music for meditation.

—*The Secret Behind Traditional Chinese Medicine,* a one-hour talk on the real power behind TCM, developed by and featuring Dr. Lu

—Taoist music meditation "The Dreamer Dreams"

For more information on programs, products and services of the Traditional Chinese Medicine World Foundation, contact:

Traditional Chinese Medicine World Foundation
396 Broadway, Suite 501
New York, NY 10013
Phone: (212) 274-1079
Fax: (212) 274-9879
www.tcmworld.org
www.breastcancer.com

Index